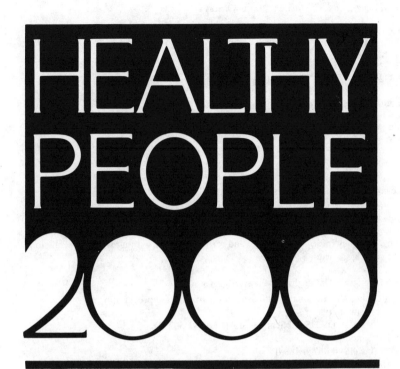

HEALTHY PEOPLE 2000

National Health Promotion and Disease Prevention Objectives

U.S. Department of Health and Human Services
Public Health Service

JONES AND BARTLETT PUBLISHERS
BOSTON   LONDON

Editorial, Sales, and Customer Service Offices

Jones and Bartlett Publishers
One Exeter Plaza
Boston, MA 02116
617-859-3900
1-800-832-0034

Jones and Bartlett Publishers International
PO Box 1498
London W6 7RS
England

Library of Congress Cataloging-in-Publication Data

Healthy people 2000 : national health promotion and disease prevention
   objectives : summary.
      p.   cm.—(DHHS publication ; no. (PHS) 91-50213)
   Includes index.
   ISBN (invalid) 0-86720-180-0
    1. Medical policy—United States. 2. Medicine, Preventive—United
States. 3. Health promotion—United States. I. Title: Healthy
people two thousand. II. Series.
   RA395.A3H436   1991   91-18617
   362.1′0973—dc20   CIP

ISBN 0-86720-180-0

The text of this document is reprinted from the original government publication, with the addition of a preface by Lawrence W. Green. The preface provides commentary on the original goals of *Healthy People 2000* and discusses how the information accepted by the government for publication departs from some of the original goals.

Reprinted from the
Department of Health and Human Services.
Publication No. (PHS) 91-50213

Healthy People 2000 is a statement of national opportunities. Although the Federal Government facilitated its development, it is not intended as a statement of Federal standards or requirements. It is the product of a national effort, involving 22 expert working groups, a consortium that has grown to include almost 300 national organizations and all the State health departments, and the Institute of Medicine of the National Academy of Sciences, which helped the U.S. Public Health Service to manage the consortium, convene regional and national hearings, and receive testimony from more than 750 individuals and organizations. After extensive public review and comment, involving more than 10,000 people, the objectives were revised and refined to produce this report.

Printed in the United States of America
95 94   10 9 8 7 6 5 4

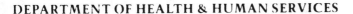
The Honorable Louis W. Sullivan
Secretary of Health and Human Services

Dear Mr. Secretary:

I am pleased to submit to you <u>Healthy People 2000: National Health Promotion and Disease Prevention Objectives</u>. This document contains a national strategy for significantly improving the health of the Nation over the coming decade. It addresses the prevention of major chronic illnesses, injuries, and infectious diseases.

The Public Health Service has served as leader, convener, and facilitator over the three-year period of this report's development. However, it can truly be labelled a national, not just a Federal, initiative to focus existing knowledge, resources, and commitment to capitalize on our opportunities to prevent premature death and needless disease and disability. Thousands of professionals from many different disciplines, as well as many health advocates and consumers, have contributed substantially to produce this set of measurable targets to be achieved by the year 2000. They have voluntarily testified at public hearings, written eloquent letters and papers, engaged in extensive reviews of draft materials, and organized and attended informational forums in support of <u>Healthy People 2000</u>. The comprehensiveness and depth of this report stand as a tribute to their commitment to better health for Americans through prevention. In addition to their contribution, Federal staff from other departments, other Operating Divisions of this Department, and the Public Health Service Agencies, have worked above and beyond the call of duty to produce this national prevention strategy. The Institute of Medicine of the National Academy of Sciences has served as an important partner in our efforts to involve a broad consortium of participants in the process. Each deserves a special note of appreciation.

I commend <u>Healthy People 2000</u> to you and through you to the American people. This set of objectives for the year 2000 makes an important, compelling point to us and to all health policy makers: we can no longer afford <u>not</u> to invest in prevention. From the perspective of avoiding human suffering as well as saving wasteful costs for treating diseases and injuries that could have been prevented, the 1990s should be the decade of prevention in the United States.

With the submission of <u>Healthy People 2000</u>, I commit the Public Health Service to work toward achievement of these objectives for the coming decade.

Sincerely yours,

James O. Mason, M.D., Dr.P.H.
Assistant Secretary for Health

Enclosure

Foreword

Americans today are taking a more active interest in their health than ever before. They are coming to realize the influence that they, themselves, can have on their own health destinies and on the overall health status of the Nation.

It wasn't always thus. Until fairly recently, we Americans gave little thought to health as a positive concept. The past 15 years or so, however, have witnessed important changes in our thinking about the protection and enhancement of personal health. Three of those changes are of great importance for the well-being of our people as we move into the final decade of this century.

First, personal responsibility, which is to say responsible and enlightened behavior by each and every individual, truly is the key to good health. Evidence of this still-evolving perspective abounds in our concern about the dangers of smoking and the abuse of alcohol and drugs; in the emphasis that we are placing on physical and emotional fitness; in our growing interest in good nutritional practices; and in our concern about the quality of our environment. We have become, in a word, increasingly health-conscious, increasingly appreciative of the extent to which our physical and emotional well-being is dependent upon measures that only we, ourselves, can affect.

We can control our health destinies in significant ways, then, but if we are to realize, fully, the benefits of assuming that control, and this is the second of the three points I would make, we must find the means of extending the benefits of good health to the most vulnerable among us.

The correlation between poor health and lower socio-economic status has been well documented, but that does not make it right or inevitable. Good health should not be seen, or, for that matter, be permitted to exist in fact, as a benefit for only those who can afford it; it should be available and accessible to every citizen.

Medical care, alone, will not eliminate the devastating impact of chronic disease on the disadvantaged, nor will it reduce, as much as we would like, the rate of infant mortality or the burden of homicide and violence or any of the other "health" problems that are borne by the poor in our society. If we are to extend the benefits of good health to all our people, it is crucial that we build in our most vulnerable populations what I have called a "culture of character," which is to say a culture, or a way of thinking and being, that actively promote responsible behavior and the adoption of lifestyles that are maximally conducive to good health. This is "prevention" in the broadest sense. It is also an absolute necessity, both because we are a humane and caring society and because, if we are to remain a vital society, we cannot afford to waste human resources. Good health must be an equal opportunity, available to all Americans.

Finally, health promotion and disease prevention comprise perhaps our best opportunity to reduce the ever-increasing portion of our resources that we spend to treat preventable illness and functional impairment. Smoking, for example, is the single most preventable cause of death and illness in this country. Smoking-related illnesses cost our health care system more than $65 billion annually.

AIDS is an almost entirely preventable disease. The cost of caring for a person with AIDS for his or her lifetime is, today, about $75,000. The annual cost of treating all diagnosed AIDS patients, about $4.3 billion this year, could climb as high as $13 billion by 1992, the Public Health Service estimates.

The yearly cost of treating alcohol and drug abuse is at least $16 billion. The total economic impact of alcohol and drug abuse, including not only treatment but premature death, accidents, crime, and lost productivity, is more than $110 billion annually.

We would be terribly remiss if we did not seize the opportunity presented by health promotion and disease prevention to dramatically cut health-care costs, to prevent the premature onset of disease and disability, and to help all Americans achieve healthier, more productive lives.

Healthy People 2000: National Health Promotion and Disease Prevention Objectives addresses these three points. It lays out a series of national opportunities. To support the development of these opportunities, a national consortium composed of nearly 300 national membership organizations and all of the State health departments joined the Department's Public Health Service to solicit and analyze comments and suggestions from people across the Nation. The Federal Departments of Agriculture, Defense, Education, Interior, Labor, and Transportation and the Environmental Protection Agency participated generously in the development of the national objectives. In regional and national hearings, the Public Health Service and its partner in this venture, the Institute of Medicine of the National Academy of Sciences, learned what people from many sectors of society consider to be the priorities for prevention in the coming decades.

This input has shaped the content of *Healthy People 2000* as it has evolved from its first drafts through extensive public review and comment to the final publication. Participants included health professionals and others in health-related industries. The Department has had the honor of serving as a convener and facilitator in developing these goals, but they truly belong to the Nation.

I commend this document for your consideration, to use as appropriate in your community. All those who participated in its development over the past three years can take pride in its clarity of vision. All of us can feel humility in the face of its monumental challenges, but we also can share a new sense of resolve to move forward to achieve a nation of healthy people.

Louis W. Sullivan, M.D.
Secretary

September 1990

Preface

With the emergence of quantified, ten-year objectives for disease prevention and health promotion in 1980[1] came new respectability and credibility to a branch of the health sciences and to health policy that previously had seemed too soft and amorphous for such specificity and concreteness. Those Objectives for 1990 and the ten-year plan that they set in motion for disease prevention and health promotion contributed enormously to a new sense of purpose and focus for public health and preventive medicine, but they had their flaws as well. The Objectives for the Year 2000 in this document build on the foundation of the Objectives for 1990 and repair many of the gaps and weaknesses in that foundation.[2]

The objectives for the previous decade were greeted in 1980 with particular skepticism by people representing the concerns of special populations, including ethnic and racial minorities and the elderly. Objectives for health and for mortality reduction in the whole population of the United States masked the considerable variations among specific population groups, particularly the vast discrepancies between rich and poor, black and white, and old and young. Many of the discrepancies in mortality and health status, some of which were glossed over by the 1990 health status objectives, reflected differences in access to health services or living conditions conducive to good health. Most of the problems selected as priorities were based on national averages, and most of the objectives pertaining to increased services and protective measures were stated generally as target averages for the nation, rather than as specific objectives for subpopulations. This problem was partially corrected soon after the 1990 Objectives were released by convening representatives of each of five special populations in separate federally-sponsored conferences. The representatives set separate health promotion priorities and identified specific barriers and resources for disease prevention and health promotion in each of these groups.[3]

From the outset of planning the Year 2000 Objectives, specificity of particular objectives for groups at higher risk has been part of the design. Major objectives in this document are delineated far more extensively than were the 1990 Objectives according to demographic and socioeconomic dimensions of risk. Chapters 2 and 3 of this document are devoted entirely to the age groups and high-risk populations. Advocacy groups for racial and ethnic populations remain disappointed that a separate category for minority-specific objectives, which was considered early in the development of the Year 2000 Objectives, did not survive in this volume. They see the need for such focus to push state and local public health agendas toward specific actions regarding minority health concerns, and to provide an authoritative source for building arguments for minority health policies. For example, the objective for restricting advertising (No. 3.15) does not explicitly target any racial or ethnic group even though these are the groups being targeted by cigarette advertising.

A second advance that the Year 2000 Objectives offer in response to criticisms of the 1990 Objectives has been the broader participation of people in setting the priorities and issues for inclusion. The process of formulating the Objectives a decade ago was largely one of building consensus among experts, professionals, and national advocacy organizations. The draft objectives were then sent out to some 3000 organizations around the country for comment and review before being put into final form. Nevertheless, the product was viewed by many as a top-down, science-driven, professionally-dominated set of objectives that gave too little weight to the social and quality-of-life concerns of people. Rather, it favored technocratic and bureaucratic criteria, such as morbidity, mortality, and cost-containment. The process of developing the Year 2000 Objectives has provided for a much more extensive and systematic pooling of perspectives from all segments of society. The Institute of Medicine of the National Academy of Sciences carried out a series of eight regional hearings on behalf of a consortium of 300 national membership organizations, the state health departments, and the federal Office of Disease Prevention and Health Promotion. At these hearings, rank and file citizens as well as local community leaders and professionals from all sectors could give testimony on issues that needed to be addressed by the Year 2000 Objectives.[4] The further comment and review process for these objectives has involved over 10,000 people.

Beyond these issues of representation in the 1990 Objectives, there were substantive concerns with the heavy reliance on leading causes of death and years of potential life lost as the criteria for setting priorities among possible categories of objectives. By permitting a wider range of criteria to give prominence to some health concerns that were of national importance, for reasons other than mortality or longevity, the Year 2000 Objectives have expanded the scope from 15 priorities to 22. Some of the new priorities identified by Chapter 8 on Educational and Community-Based Services, and Chapter 22 on Surveillance and Data Systems, were encompassed in the 1990 Objectives, but their separate identity in this document gives them greater prominence. Other new categories of objectives, such as those for the elderly, the disabled, and Chapter 6 on Mental Health clearly give greater prominence to quality-of-life and social concerns as an extension of the narrower biomedical perspective on health.

The framers of the Year 2000 Objectives continued to avoid the temptation, and the pressure from some quarters of the health services research world,[5] to include only those objectives for which there were data systems already in place to measure progress. A larger proportion of the new objectives are now more measurable than were the 1990 Objectives, thanks in part to the effect of publishing them as objectives in 1980 even though baseline measures were unavailable.[6] Development of data should follow from what is considered important, not vice versa. If the only problems that qualified for objectives were those for which data were already available, the priorities would have been quite different and, to a large degree, trivialized.

When the dust settled on the 1980s, the Objectives for the Nation in health promotion and disease prevention had proved themselves a useful guidepost for many federal agencies, state governments, and even local organizations. The federal agencies of the Public Health Service had participated actively in the formulation of the Objectives, but some might have thought the exercise would be forgotten with the arrival of the Reagan Administration in 1981. The new Assistant Secretary for Health, Edward Brandt, however, recognized the Objectives as a consensus document and not merely a Democratic Party platform. With a stroke of the pen, he issued a momentous directive that set in motion the full weight of the Objectives as official policy of the Public Health Service for the decade. He instructed the agencies of the Public Health Service to prepare their fiscal 1982 budgets using the Objectives as their justification. Thus, the Centers for Disease Control, Food and Drug Administration, the Health Resources and Services Administration, the National Institutes of Health, and the Alcohol, Drug Abuse, and Mental Health Administration all were required to link their existing programs and new budget initiatives to specific Objectives for the Nation as a basis for defending their budget requests.

State governments quickly recognized the 1990 Objectives as a template that they could use, with appropriate adaptation, for statewide health promotion and disease prevention planning. Some state health agencies, notably those in California, Colorado, Texas, and Virginia, developed their own versions of Objectives for 1990 for their individual states. Some of these developed statewide coalitions to develop the Objectives as a broad consensus process. This has provided an ongoing basis for coordination and development in these states. Some organized their monitoring and surveillance activities around a commitment to track their progress toward achievement of the Objectives for 1990. The Association of State and Territorial Health Officials used the national objectives process as a basis for promoting "The National Health Objectives Act" to support state health agencies in their implementation of the Objectives. This act was passed by the Senate but not the House in 1990. The effort did result, however, in an additional $11 million in the Prevention Block Grants to states.

At the local level, health professionals and people working on health problems in other sectors found inspiration and guidance in the Objectives for the Nation.[7] It was a greater stretch to interpolate the quantification of national objectives to the local level, but this spurred greater attention to the Model Standards for local public health agencies.[8] This document, in its first two editions in the 1980s, had a loose relationship to the Objectives for the Nation for 1990, but the third edition will have a highly integrated one-to-one correspondence between the Model Standards for local health agencies and the national Objectives for the Year 2000.[9]

Even with the improvements in the process of developing the Year 2000 Objectives, and even with the expanded content and local relevance of the objectives, other concerns will continue to dampen the wholehearted endorsement of the Objectives by some. The controversies that arose in response to the 1990 National Objectives for Health Promotion and Disease Prevention particularly raised concern among many health professionals that the Objectives would be used to cast most of the responsibility for health improvement on individuals, rather than on government. The fact that the 1990 Objectives first came to most people's attention at about the time of the arrival of the first Reagan Administration in January 1981, and the fact that the new administration embraced the Objectives while simultaneously announcing deep cuts in health services and in health protection agencies' budgets, such as those of HRSA, OSHA, and NIOSH, gave pause to those who were otherwise enthusiastic about the Objectives. The compelling rationale and statistical justification for refocusing at least some of the prevention policies toward greater emphasis on behavioral and lifestyle determinants of health (the health promotion objectives) was lost on those who viewed this refocusing as a smoke screen for the Administration's cut in health services and health protection budgets. This view was reinforced by the simultaneous development of the policies of deregulation, crippling the authority of the health protection agencies.[10] It was not the objectives themselves that aroused so much suspicion, but the political context into which they fell in 1981 following their publication in 1980.

Like the 1990 Objectives, the Year 2000 Objectives were clearly crafted to spread the burden of change among individuals, health professionals, other providers of services, schools, employers, communities, food producers and distributors, insurance companies, mass media and other industries, and government at all levels. The health promotion objectives give the impression of throwing the primary burden on individuals insofar as the risk factors for this set of objectives, more than the health protection and health services objectives, are behavioral. But the objectives themselves include these various levels of intervention, mostly under the rubric of "services and protection objectives" within each chapter of the health promotion section. The Year 2000 document states that "A supportive social environment may be the most important factor in changing behaviors that contribute to many of today's leading health threats" (p. 64). Provisions in the budgets and programs of the current federal administration, however, do not seem to provide the support or the incentives for the service providers, schools, communities, industry, or others to alter the environmental conditions that conspire against behavior conducive to health.

The immediate response to the release of the official "conference edition" of the Year 2000 Objectives at the Healthy People 2000 Conference in Washington, D. C. on September 9, 1990 was generally positive, but two criticisms were widely heard. One was that the government had made little provision for the necessary program supports, leaving the appearance of blaming the victims of poor health. The second was that they departed significantly in some instances from the objectives that had achieved consensus in the scientific, professional, and organizational review procedures. These deviations were attributable to the White House clearance procedures and were most notable in the chapters on violence control, family planning, and access to preventive health services. Examples of the differences between the consensus version of specific objectives and the edited versions after White House and OMB clearance follow.

- The original Chapter 5, originally titled "Sexual Behavior," was retitled "Family Planning" and specific objectives were altered. For example, a specific objective for achieving age-appropriate sex education in schools disappeared.

- Throughout the document, the term "comprehensive school health" was replaced with the term "quality school health," apparently to avoid any suggestion of support for sex education, school contraceptive services and other controversial subjects or services.

- The chapter on Violent and Abusive Behavior replaces the term "firearm-injury death" with the more ambiguous term "weapon-related violent death," obscuring the role of handgun control.

- The chapter on Tobacco weakened the force of objective 3.15 with the addition of a few words: "Eliminate *or severely restrict* . . . tobacco product advertising and promotion to which youth younger than age 18 *are likely to be exposed*" (italics indicating added words).

- The consensus version of objective 21.4 was "Increase to at least 60 percent the proportion of people with health insurance coverage for the screening, counseling, and immunization services recommended by the U.S. Preventive Services Task Force." The "official" version is now "Improve financing and delivery of clinical preventive services so that virtually no American has a financial barrier to receiving, at a minimum, the screening, counseling, and immunization services recommended by the U.S. Preventive Services Task force." The administration's wording avoids a commitment to providing insurance coverage and puts the burden of coverage on those delivering services.

These are noted here as a service to the good faith efforts of those who participated in the consensus development process. The need for the administration, for political reasons, to alter the specific wording in some of these is understandable, but it is also fortunate that the integrity of the consensus process can be honored in this "unofficial" publication. Staff of the Public Health Service and the Institute of Medicine and hundreds of concerned professionals and citizens around the country worked hard to produce a consensus document on Objectives for the Year 2000. Some of the credibility and acceptability this document deserves is threatened by the unseen political hand behind the revision of a few objectives. The disclaimer at the bottom of the title page, which reads like a Surgeon General's Warning, should have been sufficient for the administration to distance itself from those consensus objectives they found objectionable.

Otherwise, this document extends and improves upon the objective-setting process, providing a road map for the 1990s and a vision of public health at the beginning of the twenty-first century. William H. Foege, Executive Director of the Carter Center and former Director of CDC, called the objective-setting process, along with development of surveillance systems and the development of epidemiology, one of the three most important public health developments in this century.

Lawrence W. Green Dr.P.H.
Policy Scholar
Institute for Health Policy Studies
University of California at
San Francisco

References

[1] Public Health Service. *Promoting Health/Preventing Disease: Objectives for the Nation*. Washington, DC: U.S. Department of Health and Human Services, 1980.

[2] Green, L.W. Healthy people: The Surgeon General's Report and the prospects. Chap. 3 in W.K. McNerney, *Working for a Healthier America*. Cambridge, MA: Ballinger Publishing Co., 1980, pp. 95–110; Mason, J.O. A prevention policy framework for the nation. *Health Affairs* 9:22–29, 1990; McGinnis, J.M. Setting nationwide objectives in disease prevention and health promotion. The United States experience. In W.W. Holland, R. Detels, and G. Knox, eds. *Oxford Textbook of Public Health*. New York: Oxford University Press, 1985.

[3] Public Health Service. *Strategies for Promoting Health for Specific Populations*. Washington, DC: Office of Health Information and Health Promotion, DHHS (PHS) Pub. No. 81-50169, 1981; reprinted in *Journal of Public Health Policy* 8:369–423, 1987.

[4] Stoto, M.A., Behrens, R., and Rosemont, C., eds., *Healthy People 2000: Citizens Chart the Course*. Washington, DC: National Academy Press, 1990.

[5] Anderson, R. and Mullner, R. Assessing the health objectives of the nation. *Health Affairs* 9:152–162, 1990.

[6] Green, L.W., Wilson, R.W., and Bauer, K. Data required to measure progress on the objectives for the nation in disease prevention and health promotion. *American Journal of Public Health* 73: 18–24, 1983.

[7] McGinnis, J.M.: Setting objectives for public health in the 1990s: Experience and Prospects. *Annual Review of Public Health* 11:231–249, 1990.

[8] *Model Standards: A Guide for Community Preventive Health Services*, 2nd ed. Washington, DC: American Public Health Association, 1985.

[9] *Healthy Communities 2000: Model Standards, Guidelines for Community Attainment of Year 2000 National Health Objectives*. Washington, DC: American Public Health Association, in press.

[10] Allegrante, J.P. and Green, L.W. When health policy becomes victim blaming. *New England Journal of Medicine* 305: 1528–1529, 1981.

Contents

Part I
Healthy People 2000

Appendices

Contents of the Full Report

Part I
Healthy People 2000

Part II
National Health Promotion and Disease Prevention Objectives

Health Promotion

1. Physical Activity and Fitness
2. Nutrition
3. Tobacco
4. Alcohol and Other Drugs
5. Family Planning
6. Mental Health and Mental Disorders
7. Violent and Abusive Behavior
8. Educational and Community-Based Programs

Health Protection

9. Unintentional Injuries
10. Occupational Safety and Health
11. Environmental Health
12. Food and Drug Safety
13. Oral Health

Preventive Services

14. Maternal and Infant Health
15. Heart Disease and Stroke
16. Cancer
17. Diabetes and Chronic Disabling Conditions
18. HIV Infection
19. Sexually Transmitted Diseases
20. Immunization and Infectious Diseases
21. Clinical Preventive Services

Surveillance and Data Systems

22. Surveillance and Data Systems

Age-Related Objectives

- Children
- Adolescents and Young Adults
- Adults
- Older Adults

Special Population Objectives

- People with Low Income
- Blacks
- Hispanics
- Asians and Pacific Islanders
- American Indians and Native Americans
- People with Disabilities

Additional Appendices

D. Mortality Objectives Technical Appendix

E. Recommendations of the U.S. Preventive Services Task Force

Acronyms and Abbreviations

ADAMHA	Alcohol, Drug Abuse, and Mental Health Administration
AHCPR	Agency for Health Care Policy and Research
ATSDR	Agency for Toxic Substances and Disease Registry
CDC	Center for Disease Control
DOD	Department of Defense
DoEd	Department of Education
DOI	Department of the Interior
DOL	Department of Labor
DOT	Department of Transportation
EPA	Environmental Protection Agency
FDA	Food and Drug Administration
FSA	Family Support Administration
HCFA	Health Care Financing Administration
HRSA	Health Resources and Services Administration
IHS	Indian Health Service
NIH	National Institutes of Health
OHDS	Office of Human Development Services
PHS	Public Health Service
SSA	Social Security Administration
USDA	Department of Agriculture

Part I

Healthy People 2000

Contents

1. Introduction

The year 2000 appears ahead on the calendar of our Nation's history as a turning point. It may well be like any other year in the ongoing lives of people who inhabit this country and the world. But from the perspective of history, the year 2000 will bring to its conclusion a tumultuous century, characterized by astounding scientific achievements, devastating world wars, and explosive population growth. It will inaugurate at once a new century and a new millennium, a future so vast in its human and historic dimensions that it defies prediction while posing momentous questions about social and economic viability and human vitality in the face of a new era.

The year 2000 connotes change. Its arrival contains enough power to shape that change, motivating actions that can improve American lives. The beginning of the twenty-first century beckons both with challenge and opportunity for improved health of Americans. We began the current century with a sense of fatalism about the Nation's health problems. As we reach its conclusion, we do so with confidence in our ability to control many of the events that form our health prospects. A century of biomedical research has made available sophisticated techniques for diagnosing and intervening against disease. Scientific studies of even the last generation have revealed much about the factors that predispose to various health threats and therefore about actions that each of us can take to control our risks for disease or disability.

We have learned that a fuller measure of health, a better quality of life, is within our personal grasp. If tobacco use in this country stopped entirely today, an estimated 390,000 fewer Americans would die before their time each year. If all Americans reduced their consumption of foods high in fat to well below current levels and engaged in physical activity no more strenuous than sustained walking for 30 minutes a day, additional results of a similar magnitude could be expected. If alcohol were never carelessly used in our society, about 100,000 fewer people would die from unnecessary illness and injury. Together, deaths from these causes comprise a sizable share of the 2.1 million deaths that occur annually and are examples of the impact of personal lifestyle choices on the health destiny of individual Americans and the future of the Nation.

New knowledge has brought with it both a keen sense of potential and a keen appreciation of how far most Americans, especially those with low incomes, are from that potential. Moreover, we are already feeling the effects of momentous new issues emerging on the horizon—the aging of our society, the prohibitive costs of many of the technologies developed for diagnosing and treating disease, and the ecologic consequences of industrialization and population growth.

These problems compel careful engagement on the national agenda. This report frames the elements of that agenda from the perspective of the potential to prevent unnecessary disease and disability and to achieve a better quality of life for all Americans. It grows out of a health strategy initiated in 1979 with the publication of *Healthy People: The Surgeon General's Report on Health Promotion and Disease Prevention*[7] and expanded with publication in 1980 of *Promoting Health/Preventing Disease: Objectives for the Nation*[8], which set out an agenda for the ten years leading up to 1990.

Healthy People 2000 offers a vision for the new century, characterized by significant reductions in preventable death and disability, enhanced quality of life, and greatly reduced disparities in the health status of populations within our society. It is the product of a national effort, involving professionals and citizens, private organizations and public agencies from every part of the country. Work on the report began in 1987 with the convening of a consortium that has grown to include almost 300 national membership organizations and all the State health departments (see Appendix B). The Healthy People 2000 Consortium, facilitated by the Institute of Medicine of the National Academy of Sciences, helped the United States Public Health Service to convene 8 regional hearings and received testimony from over 750 individuals and organizations. This testimony became the primary resource material for working groups of professionals to use in crafting the health objectives. After extensive public review and comment, involving more than 10,000 people, the objectives were refined and revised to produce this report.

This report does not reflect the policies or opinions of any one organization, including the Federal government, or any one individual. It is the product of a national process. It is deliberately comprehensive in addressing health promotion and disease prevention opportunities in order to allow local communities and States to choose from among its recommendations in addressing their own highest priority needs.

The Year 2000: A Profile of The American People

Over the course of the 1990s, the profile of the American population will change. Barring unforeseeable major events, the demographic contrasts between 1990 and 2000 will be evident, if not dramatic. Based on the best available information:

- By the year 2000, the overall population of the United States will have grown about 7 percent to nearly 270 million people, with the slowest rate of growth in the Nation's history projected between 1995 and 2000.[12] Average household size is expected to decline from 2.69 in 1985 to 2.48 in 2000, with husband-wife households decreasing from 58 to 53 percent of all households.[1]

- By the year 2000, the American population will be older, continuing the aging trend of the present century, with a median age of more than 36 years, compared to 29 years in 1975. The number of children under age 5 will actually decline from more than 18 million to fewer than 17 million between 1990 and 2000. By 2000, the 35 million people over age 65 will represent about 13 percent of the population, in contrast to 8 percent in 1950. The population of the "oldest old"—those over age 85—will have increased by about 30 percent to a total of 4.6 million by 2000.[12]

- By the year 2000, the racial and ethnic composition of the American population will form a different pattern. Whites, not including Hispanic Americans, will represent a smaller proportion of the total, declining from 76 to 72 percent of the population. One particularly fast-growing population group will be Hispanics, some estimates forecasting a rise from 8 to 11.3 percent, to more than 31 million Hispanic people by 2000. Blacks will increase their proportion from 12.4 to 13.1 percent. Other racial groups, including American Indians and Alaska Natives and Asians and Pacific Islanders, will increase from 3.5 to 4.3 percent of the total.[11,12]

- By the year 2000, economic expansion will create up to 18 million new jobs, but the number of young job seekers will decline due to a shift in birth rates. Reflecting changes in racial and ethnic populations, the entry rate of blacks, Hispanics, Asians and Pacific Islanders, and American Indians and Alaska Natives into the workforce will be higher than for whites. Women of all racial and ethnic groups will be the major source of new entrants into the labor force, comprising 47 percent of the total workforce by 2000, compared to 45 percent in 1988. Half of women in the workforce will be between the ages of 35 and 54, a shift from 1986 when the majority were between 25 and 44. Between 1988 and the year 2000, white men will comprise only 25 percent of the net growth of the labor force.[4] Occupations most likely to grow include service, professional, technical, sales, and executive and management positions.

2

- By the year 2000, the American population may increase by up to 6 million people through immigration. Certain States and cities, especially those on the east and west coasts, can be expected to receive a disproportionately large number of these immigrants.[6]

While 10 years in the history of a nation seems a comparatively short time, it is long enough to alter population patterns in ways that are of great importance to current and future decision-makers seeking to design an effective program of health promotion and disease prevention. Informed estimates about the changes in households and family constellations, age groups, racial and ethnic populations, the workforce, and immigration can provide a context that is crucial to decisions and programs to achieve a nation of healthy people.

Promoting Health and Preventing Disease: Progress

Ten years is also long enough to bring about marked changes in the Nation's health (Fig. 1.1). During the 1980s, there were major declines in death rates for three of the leading causes of death among Americans: heart disease, stroke, and unintentional injuries. Infant mortality also decreased, and some childhood infectious diseases were nearly eliminated. Gains in these areas give hope that the 1990s will see more progress, especially for diseases such as cancer that have so far not declined.

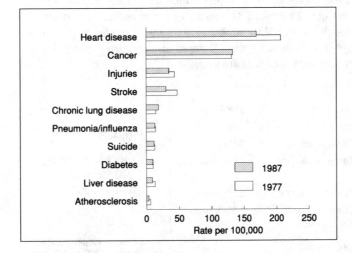

Fig. 1.1

Leading causes of death, U.S. population (age-adjusted)

Source: *Health, United States, 1989 and Prevention Profile* and National Center for Health Statistics (CDC)

Much of our progress mirrors reductions in risk factors. The more than 40-percent drop in heart disease mortality since 1970 reflects dramatic increases in high blood pressure detection and control, a decline in cigarette smoking, and increasing awareness of the role of blood cholesterol and dietary fats. The precipitous drop in stroke death rates—over 50 percent in the same period—also reflects gains in hypertension control and declines in smoking.

Unintentional injuries have declined. In the last decade and a half, traffic fatalities dropped by one-third, partly reflecting increased use of seatbelts, lower speed limits, and declines in alcohol abuse. Recent reductions in fatal occupational injuries have been facilitated by enhanced occupational safety standards. Studies are beginning to yield promising approaches to alcohol and other drug problems.

Progress has been made in the health status of children as well. In 1987, we achieved a record low rate of 10.1 infant deaths per 1,000 live births.[5] Although still higher than rates in many other developed countries, this figure represents a 65-percent decline since 1950. Preventable childhood diseases, such as mumps, measles, and rubella, are now unusual in this country due to widespread use of vaccines. Immunization levels among school children exceed 95 percent for most of these diseases.

In other areas, progress is mixed. Lung cancer deaths have increased steadily since 1960, although rates among men aged 50 and younger began to turn around in the 1980s, a sign that changes in smoking patterns are beginning to have an effect. Breast cancer death rates remain stubbornly high, as they have for 35 years, despite the fact that early detection and treatment could reduce deaths due to breast cancer by an estimated 30 percent.[10] For cervical cancer, the widespread use of Pap tests has contributed to a 73-percent reduction in death rates from the disease since 1950.

Changing trends point to still other areas that require attention. In the past decade, rising rates of syphilis and the emergence of HIV infection point to the need for new strategies to address these public health problems. Air and water quality have improved since the Environmental Protection Agency and the States began regulating them in the early 1970s. However, the last decade has seen increasing concern expressed by individuals, communities, and public agencies about toxic substances, solid waste, and global environmental change.

When taken together, the progress of the last ten years has brought the Nation a considerable distance toward the health goals set forth in *Healthy People* in 1979. That report targeted for the year 1990 a 35-percent reduction in infant mortality, a 20-percent reduction in death rates for children aged 1 through 14, a 20-percent reduction in death rates for adolescents and young adults aged 15 through 24, and a 25-percent reduction in death rates for adults aged 25 through 64. For older adults, aged 65 and older, the target was a 20-percent reduction in days of disability. Figure 1.2 summarizes progress toward these goals, as of the most recent year for which data are available.

Life Stage	1990 Target*	1987 Status
Infants	35% lower death rate	28% lower
Children	20% lower death rate	21% lower
Adolescents/ Young Adults	20% lower death rate	13% lower
Adults	25% lower death rate	21% lower
Older Adults	20% fewer days of restricted activity	17% lower

* Relative to baseline (1977 data)

Fig. 1.2

Progress toward 1990 life stage goals—1987

Source: *Health, United States, 1989* and *Prevention Profile*

A more detailed record of national efforts in health promotion and disease prevention is provided by tracking progress toward achievement of the 226 measurable objectives that were laid out in *Promoting Health/Preventing Disease: Objectives for the Nation* in 1980—objectives established to achieve the broad goals of *Healthy People*. As of 1987, it appeared that nearly half of the objectives had been achieved or were well on their way toward achievement by 1990; about one-quarter appeared unlikely to be achieved; and the status of the other quarter was uncertain because data were unavailable for tracking their progress.[5] Among the 15 priority areas that were the focus of the 1990 objectives, areas in which progress seemed to lag included pregnancy and infant health, nutrition, physical fitness and exercise, family planning, sexually transmitted diseases, and occupational safety and health. On the other hand, priority areas related to high blood pressure control, immunization, control of infectious diseases, unintentional injury prevention and control, smoking, and alcohol and drugs showed substantial progress.[5]

Healthy People: The Economics of Prevention

Despite the overall health improvements achieved as a result of preventive interventions, the Nation continues to be burdened by preventable illness, injury, and disability. In 1960, the share of the Gross National Product (GNP) going to medical services was 5 percent. It is estimated to reach nearly 12 percent in 1990.[2] Lost economic productivity attendant to illness and early death compounds the impact of this problem, so that in 1980 the total costs of illness equalled nearly 18 percent of GNP. Injury alone now costs the Nation well over $100 billion annually, cancer over $70 billion, and cardiovascular disease $135 billion.[3,9]

Sophisticated technology for the diagnosis and treatment of disease conditions has outstripped society's ability to pay for it. But many of these expenses are avoidable (Fig. 1.3). Coronary artery disease affects approximately 7 million Americans and causes about 1.5 million heart attacks and 500,000 deaths a year. The number of coronary

Condition	Overall magnitude	Avoidable intervention [1]	Cost per patient [2]
Heart disease	7 million with coronary artery disease 500,000 deaths/yr 284,000 bypass procedures/yr	Coronary bypass surgery	$30,000
Cancer	1 million new cases/yr 510,000 deaths/yr	Lung cancer treatment	$29,000
		Cervical cancer treatment	$28,000
Stroke	600,000 strokes/yr 150,000 deaths/yr	Hemiplegia treatment and rehabilitation	$22,000
Injuries	2.3 million hospitalizations/yr 142,500 deaths/yr 177,000 persons with spinal cord injuries in the United States	Quadriplegia treatment and rehabilitation	$570,000 (lifetime)
		Hip fracture treatment and rehabilitation	$40,000
		Severe head injury treatment and rehabilitation	$310,000
HIV infection	1-1.5 million infected 118,000 AIDS cases (as of Jan 1990)	AIDS treatment	$75,000 (lifetime)
Alcoholism	18.5 million abuse alcohol 105,000 alcohol-related deaths/yr	Liver transplant	$250,000
Drug abuse	Regular users: 1-3 million, cocaine 900,000, IV drugs 500,000, heroin Drug-exposed babies: 375,000	Treatment of drug-affected baby	$63,000 (5 years)
Low birth weight baby	260,000 LBWB born/yr 23,000 deaths/yr	Neonatal intensive care for LBWB	$10,000
Inadequate immunization	Lacking basic immunization series: 20-30%, aged 2 and younger 3%, aged 6 and older	Congenital rubella syndrome treatment	$354,000 (lifetime)

[1]Examples (other interventions may apply).
[2]Representative first-year costs, except as noted. Not indicated are nonmedical costs, such as lost productivity to society.

Fig. 1.3

Costs of treatment for selected preventable conditions

Source: Data compiled from various sources by the Office of Disease Prevention and Health Promotion

bypass procedures performed each year is approaching 300,000, each *one* of these procedures at a cost of approximately $30,000. A representative cost for treating a single case of lung cancer is $29,000 and $28,000 for invasive cervical cancer. A liver transplant for alcoholic cirrhosis can cost $250,000 or more. The lifetime treatment costs per patient are $570,000 for quadriplegia from a spinal cord injury, $354,000 for congenital rubella syndrome, and $75,000 for Acquired Immunodeficiency Syndrome (AIDS). Yet virtually all of these conditions are preventable. Mobilizing the considerable energies and creativity of the Nation in the interest of disease prevention and health promotion is an economic imperative.

Healthy People 2000: The Challenge and Goals

The Nation has within its power the ability to save many lives lost prematurely and needlessly. Implementation of what is already known about promoting health and preventing disease is the central challenge of *Healthy People 2000*. But *Healthy People 2000* also challenges the Nation to move beyond merely saving lives. The health of a people is measured by more than death rates. Good health comes from reducing unnecessary suffering, illness, and disability. It comes as well from an improved quality of life. Health is thus best measured by citizens' sense of well-being. The health of a Nation is measured by the extent to which the gains are accomplished for all the people.

The challenge of *Healthy People 2000* is to use the combined strength of scientific knowledge, professional skill, individual commitment, community support, and political will to enable people to achieve their potential to live full, active lives. It means preventing premature death and preventing disability, preserving a physical environment that supports human life, cultivating family and community support, enhancing each individual's inherent abilities to respond and to act, and assuring that all Americans achieve and maintain a maximum level of functioning.

The purpose of *Healthy People 2000* is to commit the Nation to the attainment of three broad goals that will help bring us to our full potential (Fig. 1.4). We have a broad array of opportunities to achieve our goals. This report presents many of these opportunities in the form of measurable targets, or objectives, to be achieved by the year 2000, organized into 22 priority areas. The first 21 of these areas are grouped into three broad categories: health promotion; health protection; and preventive services (Fig. 1.5).

- **Increase the span of healthy life for Americans**
- **Reduce health disparities among Americans**
- **Achieve access to preventive services for all Americans**

Fig. 1.4

Healthy People 2000 Goals

Health promotion strategies are those related to individual lifestyle—personal choices made in a social context—that can have a powerful influence over one's health prospects. These priorities include physical activity and fitness, nutrition, tobacco, alcohol and other drugs, family planning, mental health and mental disorders, and violent and abusive behavior. Educational and community-based programs can address lifestyle in a crosscutting fashion.

Health protection strategies are those related to environmental or regulatory measures that confer protection on large population groups. These strategies address issues such as unintentional injuries, occupational safety and health, environmental health, food and drug safety, and oral health. Interventions applied to address these issues are generally

Health Promotion
1. Physical Activity and Fitness
2. Nutrition
3. Tobacco
4. Alcohol and Other Drugs
5. Family Planning
6. Mental Health and Mental Disorders
7. Violent and Abusive Behavior
8. Educational and Community-Based Programs

Health Protection
9. Unintentional Injuries
10. Occupational Safety and Health
11. Environmental Health
12. Food and Drug Safety
13. Oral Health

Preventive Services
14. Maternal and Infant Health
15. Heart Disease and Stroke
16. Cancer
17. Diabetes and Chronic Disabling Conditions
18. HIV Infection
19. Sexually Transmitted Diseases
20. Immunization and Infectious Diseases
21. Clinical Preventive Services

Surveillance and Data Systems
22. Surveillance and Data Systems

Age-Related Objectives
Children
Adolescents and Young Adults
Adults
Older Adults

Fig. 1.5

Healthy People 2000
Priority Areas

not exclusively protective in nature—there may be a substantial health promotion element as well—but the principal approaches involve a communitywide rather than individual focus.

Preventive services include counseling, screening, immunization, or chemoprophylactic interventions for individuals in clinical settings. Priority areas for these strategies include maternal and infant health, heart disease and stroke, cancer, diabetes and chronic disabling conditions, HIV infection, sexually transmitted diseases, and infectious diseases. Crosscutting professional and access considerations in the delivery of clinical preventive services are also addressed.

A special category has been established for surveillance and data systems. Given the centrality of monitoring progress toward the stated targets in the overall approach of *Healthy People 2000*, the integrity of our data collection efforts at every level is critical. Objectives have therefore been established to improve those efforts.

Finally, because issues and approaches vary by age, chapters are included for each of four age groups: children, adolescents and young adults, adults, and older adults. Objectives related to each of these age groups are found throughout the priority areas. To give them special emphasis, some of the key targets have been collected and presented according to these four ages.

The full set of objectives with commentary is presented as Part II of *Healthy People 2000*. The material presented here in Part I defines the overall national agenda and outlines goals, objectives, and strategies for change. Chapter 2 of Part I reviews the challenges for people in various age groups. Chapter 3 addresses high risk populations. Chapter 4 presents the broad goals. Chapter 5 gives synopses of each of the priority areas with selected examples of the objectives addressed. Chapter 6 reviews the challenge for implementation for various groups throughout the Nation.

The last chapter deserves special comment. *Healthy People 2000* uses the three approaches of health promotion, health protection, and preventive services as organizing categories, but running through the priority areas and the objectives is a common theme of shared responsibility for carrying out this national agenda. Achievement of the agenda depends heavily on changes in individual behaviors. It requires use of legislation, regulation, and social sanctions to make the social and physical environment a healthier place to live. It calls on medical and health professionals to prevent, not just to treat, the diseases and conditions that result in premature death and chronic disability. All are necessary. None is sufficient alone to achieve *Healthy People 2000*'s goals and objectives.

The challenge spelled out in *Healthy People 2000* calls upon communities to translate national objectives into State and local action. To accomplish this, a new edition of Model Standards—*Healthy Communities 2000: Model Standards, Guidelines for Attainment of Year 2000 Objectives for the Nation*—provides a flexible planning tool to enable communities to share in the various efforts necessary to attain these objectives. The volume covers the priority areas of *Healthy People 2000* and includes all of the national objectives that call for action at the community level. It offers community implementation strategies for putting the objectives of *Healthy People 2000* into practice and encourages communities to establish achievable community health targets.

References

[1] Bureau of the Census. *Projections of the Numbers of Households and Families: 1986 to 2000*. Washington, DC: U.S. Department of Commerce, 1986.

[2] Health Care Financing Administration, Office of the Actuary. Expenditures and percent of gross national product for national health expenditures, by private and public funds, hospital care, and physician services; calendar years 1960-87. *Health Care Financing Review* 10:2, Winter 1988.

[3] Hodgson, T.A., and Rice, D.P. Economic impact of cancer in the United States. In: Schottenfeld, D., ed. *Cancer Epidemiology and Prevention*. Chapter 13, in press.

[4] Kutscher, R.E. Projections 2000: Overview and implications of the projections to 2000. *Monthly Labor Review* September, 1987.

[5] National Center for Health Statistics. *Health, United States, 1989 and Prevention Profile*. DHHS Pub. No. (PHS)90-1232. Hyattsville, MD: U.S. Department of Health and Human Services, 1990.

[6] Passel, J.E., and Woodrow, K.A. "Immigration to the United States." Paper presented to the Census Table, August 1986.

[7] Public Health Service. *Healthy People: Surgeon General's Report on Health Promotion and Disease Prevention*. Washington, DC: U.S. Department of Health and Human Services, 1979.

[8] Public Health Service. *Promoting Health/Preventing Disease: Objectives for the Nation*. Washington, DC: U.S. Department of Health and Human Services, 1980.

[9] Rice, D.P.; MacKenzie, E.J.; Jones, A.S.; Kaufman, S.R.; deLissovoy, G.V.; Max, W.; McLoughlin, E.; Miller, T.R.; Robertson, L.S.; Salkever, D.S.; and Smith, G.S. *Cost of Injury in the United States: A Report to Congress, 1989*. San Francisco, CA: Institute for Health and Aging, University of California and Injury Prevention Center, The Johns Hopkins University, 1989.

[10] Shapiro, S.; Venet, W.; Strax, L.; and Roeser, R. Selection, Followup, and Analysis in the Health Insurance Plan Study: A Randomized Trial With Breast Cancer Screening. *National Cancer Institute Monographs* 67:65-74, 1985.

[11] Spencer, G. Projections of the Hispanic Population: 1983-2080. *Current Population Reports, Population Estimates and Projections*. Series P-25, No. 995. Washington, DC: U.S. Department of Commerce, Bureau of the Census, 1986.

[12] Spencer, G. Projections of the population of the United States, by age, sex, and race: 1988 to 2080. *Current Population Reports, Population Estimates and Projections*. Series P-25, No. 1018. Washington, DC: U.S. Department of Commerce, Bureau of the Census, 1989.

2. The Nation's Health: Age Groups

Responding effectively to the health challenges of the 1990s will require a clear understanding of the health-related threats and opportunities facing all Americans. One way to grasp the dimensions and the realities of the tasks laid out in this report is to consider the special problems of infants, children, adolescents and young adults, adults, and older adults. The health profiles of these age groups can help us remember that the improvements envisioned here are not generalizations about the population, but prescriptions for healthier lives for each of us—newborn babies, boys and girls, teenagers and young people, women and men, and people in their later years.

Infants

One of the most heartening indicators of our Nation's improvement in health during the 20th century has been the steady decline in the infant mortality rate. Between 1950 and 1987, the infant mortality rate in the United States dropped from 29.2 per 1,000 live births to 10.1. Eight years after *Healthy People* (1979) posed the challenge of a 35-percent reduction in infant mortality by 1990, we had achieved a reduction of 28 percent in that rate.[38]

Yet comparison of even our 1987 rate of infant mortality with that of other industrialized nations demonstrates the continued importance of efforts in this regard. Moreover, the continuing disparities between minority and majority populations represent a major health challenge. In 1987, the mortality rate for black infants was still over twice that of whites, and rates for some American Indian tribes and for Puerto Ricans were also considerably higher than for white infants.[38]

Infant mortality rates provide a summary measure of the effects of major health threats to the developing fetus and newborn baby. But for every 10 babies who die, 990 live. Some of those who live have been harmed, often permanently, by unhealthy beginnings. The quality, not just the quantity, of their lives is a function of health during both the prenatal and infant periods.

Technology has contributed significantly to the improved prospects for infant survival over the past several decades. Neonatal intensive care, new surgical techniques, and other medical interventions save lives and even overcome conditions that formerly guaranteed life-long disability. But opportunities for primary prevention offer new frontiers for improving infant health in the coming years. Some opportunities will result from breakthroughs in understanding the genetic origins of human diseases; most will be in areas of personal lifestyle and use of existing health interventions.

Major Health Concerns

No period of life is more important to good health than the months before birth. The prenatal period can be the starting time for good health or it may be the beginning of a lifetime of illness and shortened life expectancy. Each year in the United States, nearly 39,000 babies—about 1 percent of those born—die before the age of one, two-thirds during their first month.[38] Four causes account for more than half of all infant deaths: disorders relating to low birth weight, congenital anomalies, sudden infant death syndrome (SIDS), and respiratory distress syndrome (Fig. 2.1).

Low birth weight (less than 2,500 grams) occurs in about 7 percent of all live births and is the greatest single hazard to infant health.[38] This dangerous condition has been linked to several preventable risks, including lack of prenatal care, maternal smoking, use of

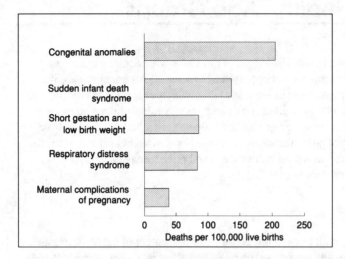

Fig. 2.1

Leading causes of
infant mortality
(1987)

Source: *Health, United
States, 1989 and Preven-
tion Profile*

alcohol and other drugs, and pregnancy before age 18. Approximately three-quarters of deaths in the first month and 60 percent of all infant deaths occurred among low-birth-weight infants. Low socioeconomic and educational levels are often associated with low birth weight. Black infants are more than twice as likely as white babies to be born weighing less than 2,500 grams.[38]

Very low birth weight (less than 1,500 grams) is associated with 40 percent of all infant deaths. Very low birth weight declined slightly from 1970 to 1981 but rose by about 0.9 percent per year from 1981 to 1986.[38] Low-birth-weight babies are nearly twice as likely to have severe developmental delay or congenital anomalies.[68] These babies are also at a significantly greater risk of such long-term disabilities as cerebral palsy, autism, mental retardation, and vision and hearing impairments, and other developmental disabilities.

Congenital anomalies (birth defects) most likely to be lethal include malformations of the brain and spine, heart defects, and combinations of several malformations. Infant mortality from congenital anomalies has been declining, although the last decade has seen slight increases in the incidence of some birth defects. In 1985, about 11,000 babies were born with moderate to severe impairments.[40] Congenital anomalies, when they do not result in death, may cause disability. One-fourth of all congenital anomalies are caused by genetic factors, suggesting a need for preconception genetic counseling for both men and women. Environmental hazards and alcohol use during pregnancy are other important factors. Fetal alcohol syndrome (FAS) affects as many as 1 to 3 infants per 1,000 live births.[38] In some populations, the incidence is higher. A similar syndrome has been observed in babies born to drug-addicted mothers.

After the first month of life, sudden infant death syndrome (SIDS) is the leading cause of infant mortality, accounting for about one-third of all deaths in this period.[59] The causes of SIDS are not known, but risk factors include maternal smoking and drug use, teenage birth, and infections late in pregnancy. Infants born to families with a history of SIDS are also at risk.

Respiratory distress syndrome occurs primarily in premature babies whose lungs are not fully developed. Therefore, risk factors for respiratory distress syndrome include those for prematurity.

Increasing rates of HIV infection and cocaine addiction in newborns are also of concern. By January 1990, more than 2,000 babies had been born with HIV infection, and some hospitals from urban communities reported rates of cocaine-addicted babies as high as 20 percent.[14] The long term consequences of these alarming trends are inestimable.

Maternal Factors

Several major maternal risk factors are associated with low birth weight, as well as with other major causes of infant death and disability, including:

- Cigarette smoking;

- Alcohol and other drug use;

- Age;

- Nutrition;

- Socioeconomic status;

- Environmental hazards.

An estimated 25 percent of pregnant women smoke throughout their pregnancies.[66] There is some evidence that pregnant women are quitting smoking and that smoking prevalence during pregnancy is decreasing for some but not all groups. Women in the lowest age and socioeconomic groups have the highest likelihood of smoking during pregnancy.[32] Maternal cigarette smoking has been linked with from 20 to 30 percent of all low-birth-weight births in the United States.[33] If all pregnant women refrained from smoking, fetal and infant deaths would be reduced by approximately 10 percent, saving about 4,000 infants per year.

Heavy alcohol consumption during pregnancy is associated with increased risk for fetal alcohol syndrome, including growth retardation, facial malformations, mental retardation, and central nervous system dysfunctions. A safe amount of alcohol consumption during pregnancy has not been documented; however, adverse effects are associated primarily with heavy consumption during the early months of pregnancy.

The effects of maternal drug use on pregnancy outcome have not been fully explored. Studies of the effects of maternal drug abuse are hampered by difficulties in distinguishing effects of drug exposure from those resulting from inadequate prenatal care or poor maternal health and nutrition. However, low birth weight and prematurity are the most serious known consequences of maternal illicit drug use. Risks due to maternal drug abuse are heightened by lack of prenatal care. Between 50 and 75 percent of substance-abusing women receive little or no prenatal care.[30] Reliable data on the prevalence of substance abuse by pregnant women is also difficult to obtain. Extrapolations of local studies suggest that mothers of as many as 10 percent of babies born each year have used one or more illicit substances during their pregnancy.[14,15,25]

Both pregnant women and newborn infants are particularly vulnerable to poor nutrition. Women who gain less than 21 pounds during pregnancy are more than twice as likely to deliver low-birth-weight infants than those who gain more.[71] Nutrition is also vital to growth and development of infants, including brain function. For most mothers, breastfeeding is an ideal way of nurturing their infants.

Maternal age is a risk factor at both ends of the childbearing years: under age 17 and over age 40. Teenage women, more than a million of whom become pregnant each year in the United States, are at particular risk of having low-birth-weight babies.[58] Birth rates for women aged 15 through 19 are virtually unchanged since 1980, remaining at more than 50 live births per 1,000 women.[2] Infants born to women over age 40 experience higher rates of congenital anomalies, such as Downs Syndrome.

Women with less than 12 years of education, an important element of socioeconomic status, are about 70 percent more likely to give birth to a low-birth-weight baby or experience an infant death than women with more than 12 years of education.[31] Similarly, poor pregnancy outcomes have been linked to other indicators of lower socioeconomic status such as lack of health insurance and poor nutrition.

Congenital anomalies may be caused by environmental factors such as viruses, chemicals, and radiation. Toxic substances can affect the fetus directly, through exposure of the mother, and indirectly, by altering maternal and paternal germ cell chromosomes. Industrial toxins, such as lead, vinyl chloride, and hydrocarbons, may affect workers in industrial plants. The reproductive effects of workplace toxins, however, are still uncertain and controversial.

Prenatal Care

Numerous studies have demonstrated that early and comprehensive prenatal care reduces rates of infant death and low birth weight. An expectant mother with no prenatal care is three times as likely to have a low-birth-weight baby. The effect of early prenatal care is especially evident in studies of high-risk groups, such as adolescents and poor women.[27,58] About 76 percent of women receive prenatal care, but rates are considerably lower for many minority groups.[73]

The 1970s saw significant increases in early prenatal care, especially in groups with the lowest levels of care. Since 1980, however, the proportion of women who begin prenatal care in the first 3 months of pregnancy has reached a plateau among all racial and ethnic groups.[38]

Prenatal care can save money. The Office of Technology Assessment has studied the potential effectiveness of prenatal care for all pregnant women living in poverty. Its findings indicate that for every instance of low birth weight averted by prenatal care, the United States health care system saves between $14,000 and $30,000 in health care costs associated with this condition.[58]

Children

The health profile of American children has shifted markedly in the past 40 years. Once dominated by the threat of major infectious diseases, such as polio, diphtheria, scarlet fever, pneumonia, measles, and whooping cough, today, widespread immunization has virtually eliminated many of these diseases. Others are in steep decline.

Between 1977 and 1987, the rate of childhood deaths declined 21 percent, exceeding the 1990 target set in *Healthy People*. Unintentional injuries have now replaced infectious diseases as the cause of greatest concern for the health of children. But even for the leading cause of injury-related deaths among children—motor vehicle crashes—heartening progress has occurred. Since 1970, the rate of childhood deaths from motor vehicle crashes has declined 41 percent for children aged 1 through 4, and 31 percent for those aged 5 through 14, primarily due to the use of car seats and seatbelts.[38] Other causes of injury-related deaths among children—drowning, falls, poisoning, fires—have also declined as a result of improved protections, with the sole exception of child homicide.

Several threats to children's health are associated with low socioeconomic status. Mental retardation, learning disorders, emotional and behavioral problems, and vision and speech impairments all appear to be more prevalent among children living in poverty, often in inner cities, than among those at higher socioeconomic levels.[62] An accurate profile of the health of U.S. children, therefore, must go beyond mortality and morbidity data. It must also consider emotional, psychological, and learning problems, the social and environmental risks to which they are related, and the total costs to the Nation.

12

Major Health Concerns

The leading cause of death in childhood—unintentional injuries—not only accounts for the most deaths but also is among the most preventable (Fig. 2.2). Other major, preventable problems include homicide, suicide, child abuse and neglect, developmental problems, and lead poisoning.

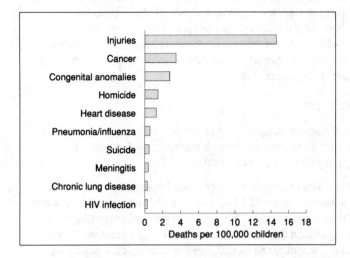

Fig. 2.2

Leading causes of death for children aged 1 through 14 (1987)

Source: National Center for Health Statistics (CDC)

Nearly half of all childhood deaths are due to unintentional injuries, and about half of these stem from motor vehicle crashes. Declines in childhood deaths from motor vehicle crashes are due in part to increasing use of child safety seats and safer automobile design. In one of the major public health successes of the decade, all 50 States now require safety restraints for young children, contributing to a 36-percent decline in motor vehicle fatalities in this age group between 1980 and 1984.[47] However, many States still do not mandate child restraints for children over age 5, and in some States there is no requirement after age 3 or 4. Furthermore, although studies suggest that 4 out of 5 passengers under age 5 now use occupant protection systems, many of the child safety seats in use have been found to be either not attached to the car seat or attached incorrectly.[48]

Drownings and fires account for most other injury-related deaths among children. Drownings are most frequent in swimming pools and home spas among children under 5. Household fires are a particular risk to children because they have more difficulty escaping than adults and are less likely to survive fire-related injuries. Deaths from fires are often due to asphyxiation and traumatic injuries, as well as burns. Children under age 5 who live in substandard housing without smoke detectors are at special risk.[24]

Injuries from falls and poisonings are not major causes of death in children but do cause many nonfatal injuries. Playground equipment and upper-story windows are frequently implicated in fall-related injuries in children.

Many injuries can be and are being prevented. During the last decade, improved safety measures have reduced fatalities. These measures include swimming pool and spa covers and childproof enclosures; child-resistant packaging for prescription drugs and some other hazardous materials; safer playground equipment; and smoke detectors. All of these, plus increased public awareness of injuries and their prevention, have helped save lives, and their wider use could save many more.

Some infections and respiratory illnesses remain problems for children. For example, influenza and other respiratory problems are the chief illness-related reasons that children miss school. In addition, the increased number of reports of asthma among children, especially those living in cities, has raised concern in recent years.[38]

Violence toward children has become of increasing concern as an American health issue, with rapidly rising rates of reported cases of child deaths due to violence. The periodic Study of National Incidence of Child Abuse and Neglect estimated that, in 1986, nearly 2 percent of children—or more than 1,000,000—were demonstrably harmed by abuse or neglect. The most common kind of abuse identified was physical, followed by emotional and sexual; the most common kind of neglect was educational, followed by physical and emotional. Substantial increases in reported physical and sexual abuse cases have occurred since 1980, but the 1986 study concluded that this was due more to improved reporting, reflecting greater public and professional awareness of the problem, than to an actual increase in child abuse. On the other hand, the study also demonstrated that many incidents of child maltreatment still go unreported.[75]

Developmental Problems

Psychological, emotional, and learning disorders are on the rise among children, as are chronic physical conditions such as hearing and speech impairment. Low-income children are at a significantly higher risk for such problems.[62]

One contributor to developmental problems in children is lead poisoning. In 1984, an estimated 3,000,000 children between 6 months and 5 years of age had blood lead levels above 15 µg/dL and 250,000 had levels above 25 µg/dL, making lead poisoning one of the Nation's most prevalent childhood threats. Severe lead poisoning can lead to profound mental retardation, coma, seizures, and death. Even low levels of exposure can impair central nervous system function, causing delayed cognitive development, hearing problems, growth retardation, and metabolic disorders.[1] Reduced lead in gasoline, air, and food, and reduced industrial emissions have produced lower mean blood lead levels nationwide. Nevertheless, homes and play areas, particularly in substandard housing areas, remain a significant source of this toxin in children's blood. The chief sources of lead exposure are thought to be old flaking lead-based paint, dust, and soil.

Healthy Child Development

Childhood is the prime time of human development. This is no less true for development of good health than it is for social, educational, emotional, and moral development. It may be easier to prevent the initiation of some behaviors, such as smoking and alcohol and drug abuse, than to intervene once they have become established. Likewise, it may be easier to establish healthful habits, such as those related to basic hygiene and those related to dietary and physical activity patterns, during childhood than later in life. Childhood is the opportune period for such healthy development.

Early use of tobacco, alcohol, and marijuana is associated with alcohol and other drug abuse later in adolescence or adulthood.[17] While most smokers start when they are young teenagers, many start even earlier. About one-quarter of high school seniors who have ever smoked report that they smoked their first cigarette by grade 6, over half by grades 7 or 8, and three-quarters by grade 9. Although cigarette smoking is declining among all age groups, those who do smoke are starting at younger ages. A wide array of factors promote smoking by children, including peer pressure, parental smoking behavior, lack of knowledge and understanding of health consequences, advertising and promotion, and the easy availability of cigarettes in unsupervised vending machines.[57]

Although the average age of first use of alcohol and marijuana is 13, pressure to begin use starts at even younger ages. Elementary school students report peer pressure to try beer, wine, and distilled spirits. Moreover, 26 percent of 4th graders and 40 percent of 6th graders reported that many of their peers had tried beer, wine, distilled spirits, or wine coolers.[51]

Lifetime diet and exercise patterns may also be established in childhood. Fat makes up more than 36 percent of calories in the average American diet, a figure that is too high according to most experts. It is recommended that children over 2, as well as adults, reduce that figure to no more than 30 percent and that saturated fats be reduced to less than 10 percent of calories. Exercise habits established in childhood may help in maintaining a physically active lifestyle throughout adolescence and adulthood. Both moderate and vigorous physical activity on a regular basis help promote overall fitness and control weight. In 1984, a little more than two-thirds of children aged 10 through 17 engaged regularly in vigorous physical activity.[72] A comparison of body composition among children between 1965 and 1985 showed a steady increase in skinfold thicknesses, a measure of body fat.

Most schools provide some health education, although the amount and content vary among States and school districts. According to recent data:

- 75 percent of school districts have antismoking education in elementary schools;[54]

- 63 percent of school districts and private schools provide some instruction concerning alcohol and other drugs and 39 percent provide related counseling;[64]

- 12 States require nutrition education from preschool through grade 12;[4]

- 32 percent of children in grades 1 through 6 and 44 percent of those in grades 7 through 9 participate in daily physical education programs, but only 1 State requires daily physical education from kindergarten through grade 12;[72]

- 25 States require comprehensive school health education programs and 9 States recommend that local school districts implement such programs.[18]

Appropriate educational strategies vary according to community and age group, but age-appropriate health education curricula can change attitudes and behavior.

Schools can also be used to facilitate children's access to basic health services. Although the traditional childhood infectious diseases have declined steeply since vaccines became available, immunization is still incomplete. Better school-based programs, information for the public, and more immunization education for physicians and health professionals are needed.

Improving the health of American children requires a wide range of social and economic interventions. For example, more and better preschool education for disadvantaged children and children with disabilities could help to detect and prevent developmental problems. Educational and support programs for parents in high-risk environments hold promise for reducing child abuse and other health problems, such as lead poisoning. The complex developmental problems besetting children in these environments demand concerted efforts by many different sectors of society. Primary care health providers, social service professionals, health educators, housing officials, community groups, and concerned individuals can each make a difference in the health of American children.

Adolescents and Young Adults

The years from 15 through 24 are a time of changing health hazards. Caught up in change and experimentation, young people also develop behaviors that may become permanent. Attitudes and patterns related to diet, physical activity, tobacco use, safety, and sexual behavior may persist from adolescence into adulthood.

The dominant preventable health problems of adolescents and young adults fall into two major categories: injuries and violence that kill and disable many before they reach age 25 and emerging lifestyles that affect their health many years later.

Two major causes of death in older age groups, heart disease and cancer, have declined sharply among adolescents since 1950—heart disease by 60 percent and cancer by 40 percent.[38] Although they are still important threats in this age group, these diseases are overshadowed by the three leading causes of death: unintentional injuries, homicide, and suicide (Fig. 2.3).

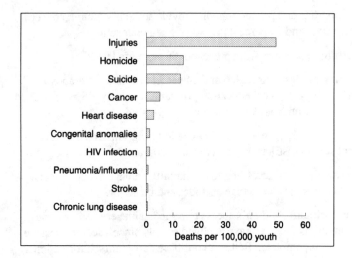

Fig. 2.3

Leading causes of death for youth aged 15 through 24 (1987)

Source: *Monthly Vital Statistics Report*, Supplement, September 26, 1989

Motor Vehicle Crash Injuries

Unintentional injuries account for about half of all deaths among people aged 15 through 24; three-quarters of these deaths involve motor vehicles. More than half of all fatal motor vehicle crashes among people in this age group involve alcohol. Young white men had the highest death rates for motor vehicle crashes in 1987, at 59 per 100,000. The rate for young black men was much lower: 36 per 100,000. The rate was lower yet for women of both races.[38]

Motor vehicle crash deaths decreased in this age group in the early 1980s, possibly because of the raised minimum drinking age in many States and decreasing alcohol use. The recent trend, however, is upward.[38] The raised speed limit on rural interstate highways may be a factor in this trend. Further, nearly 60 percent of 8th and 10th graders reported not using seatbelts on their most recent ride.[5]

Homicide and Suicide

Homicide is the second leading cause of death among all adolescents and young adults, and it is the number one cause among black youth. The homicide rate for young black men increased by 40 percent between 1984 and 1987 to nearly 86 per 100,000, more than 7 times the rate for young white men. Race, however, appears not to be as important a risk factor for violent death as socioeconomic status. Racial differences in homicide rates are significantly reduced when socioeconomic factors are taken into account.

As with motor vehicle accidents, about half of all homicides are associated with alcohol use. Nationwide, 10 percent are drug-related, but in many cities this rate is substantially higher. Over half of all homicide victims are relatives or acquaintances of the perpetrators. Most are killed with firearms.[11]

Suicide is the second leading cause of death among young white men aged 15 to 24, and rates continue to climb. From 1950 to 1987 the death rate from suicide in this group increased from under 7 to about 23 per 100,000 population. The rate of suicides among black adolescents and young adults is half of that among whites. White men between 20 and 24 years of age are more likely to commit suicide than their counterparts aged 15 through 19, but the gap between these two groups is narrowing. In general, suicides have decreased among older youth and increased among the younger cohort.[35]

Both white and black young women have relatively low suicide rates (4.7 and 2.3 respectively in 1987), although young women attempt suicide unsuccessfully approximately three times more often than young men.[35] As is the case with homicides, 60 percent of suicides among adolescents and young adults are committed with firearms.

Tobacco, Alcohol, and Drugs

Many of the most important risk factors for chronic disease in later years also have their roots in youthful behavior. The earlier cigarette smoking begins, for example, the less likely the smoker is to quit. Three-fourths of high school seniors who smoke report that they smoked their first cigarette by grade 9. Young people, especially teenage girls, are taking up smoking at younger ages. The age of initiation for regular smoking among females is now roughly the same as for males.[57]

In 1976, about 29 percent of high school seniors reported daily smoking. Between 1977 and 1981, the rate of smoking dropped to 19 percent and has since leveled off. The annual surveys of high school seniors do not gather information on school dropouts—about 15 percent of white youths and 23 percent of black youths[9]—among whom smoking is more prevalent.[61] But data for young adults aged 20 through 24 have shown a continued steady decline in cigarette smoking for young men and a recent equivalent decline for young women.

The use of snuff and chewing tobacco has increased dramatically in recent years among teenage boys. Between 1970 and 1986, snuff use increased fifteen-fold and chewing tobacco use increased fourfold among young men aged 17 through 19. In 1987, the prevalence of smokeless tobacco use among young men aged 18 through 24 was nearly 9 percent. Among younger adolescent boys aged 12 through 17, nearly 7 percent had used some form of smokeless tobacco within the last month.[65]

Alcohol consumption among teenagers and young adults is declining slowly, but it remains a major problem for both. It is a particular problem among school dropouts. Alcohol is a major contributor to both motor vehicle crashes and violence, two of the leading causes of death and disability among young people. In 1989, about 60 percent of high school seniors reported drinking alcohol in the previous month, while 33 percent reported occasions of heavy drinking—having five or more drinks on one occasion in the last 2 weeks; both figures represented slight declines from 1988 survey results.[49]

Alcohol use is also prevalent both among younger teenagers and those who are beyond high school age. In a 1987 national survey, 28 percent of 8th graders and 38 percent of 10th graders reported occasions of heavy drinking.[5] Among young people aged 18 to 24, drinking is more prevalent than in any other age group. In 1988, more than 65 percent of this group reported alcohol use during the past month.[38]

The use of illicit drugs among adolescents has been declining since the late 1970s, at least among young people who remain in school.[51] The number of high school seniors reporting illicit drug use reached a record low of about 20 percent in 1989, indicating a 50 percent drop in drug use over the last decade. Marijuana use, which peaked in 1978 at 37 percent, was down to 17 percent at the close of the 1980s. Only 3 percent of the class of 1989 reported using cocaine at least once in the last 30 days, a significant decline from the 1985 peak of 6.7 percent. Use of crack cocaine declined slightly, from 1.6 percent of high school seniors in 1988 to 1.4 percent in 1989. A more dramatic drop occurred the previous year, however, when the percentage of seniors who reported having ever used crack declined by 20 percent.[49]

Experimentation with illicit drugs often starts early. For example, in a 1987 survey of 8th and 10th graders, 6 and 10 percent, respectively, reported using marijuana in the preceding month. Slightly smaller percentages reported trying cocaine, and about a third of these had tried crack. Students' attitudes toward drugs, as toward alcohol, underwent a change during the 1980s.[5]

Sexual Behavior

An estimated 78 percent of adolescent girls and 86 percent of adolescent boys have engaged in sexual intercourse by age 20.[53,69] The risks of early sexual activity include not only unwanted pregnancy, but also infection by sexually transmitted diseases. Of the approximately 1.1 million girls aged 15 through 19 who become pregnant each year, an estimated 84 percent did not intend pregnancies. Many of these young women face serious health and psychosocial risks. Teenage mothers are more likely than others not to finish school, to be unemployed, to have low-birth-weight babies, and to lack parental skills.[23,29]

Clearly for young adolescents the most effective means of preventing possible physical and psychosocial problems related to sexual intercourse is to delay sexual activity. But, teenage sexual activity is a complex issue, embedded in family, social, and economic factors. Interventions to prevent associated negative health outcomes must address those factors if they are to succeed. For example, it has become clear to many that such interventions cannot be successful without the full support and involvement of parents and others who serve in advisory and role-model capacities with teenagers.

Lifelong Health Habits

It is important for adolescents and young adults to lay the foundation for chronic disease prevention by the promotion and maintenance of healthy lifestyles. The adoption of low-fat and low-salt dietary patterns are important for many people in the prevention of coronary heart disease and high blood pressure, and certain cancers. Further, the adoption of dietary and physical activity habits that will reduce the onset of obesity will help reduce the likelihood of coronary heart disease, diabetes, and high blood pressure. The case of physical activity is important because as students leave the school setting they lose the physical and social supports and incur time constraints that can result in decreased levels of physical activity. It is especially important for adolescents and young adults to recognize the importance of regular light to moderate physical activity in the prevention of weight gain associated with leaving the high school setting.

Although the 1980s brought some improvements in the health status of adolescents and young adults, many other young people still must confront a constellation of problems, including alcohol and other drug abuse, school failure, delinquency, peer group violence, and unwanted pregnancy. While education about risks to health is important, programs for adolescents and young adults must go beyond education to include in-depth counseling and support. Especially for youth in high-risk environments, comprehensive programs are needed to provide positive alternatives to alcohol and other drug abuse, teenage pregnancy, and lifestyles conducive to violence.

Adults

Perhaps more than any other age group, adults have the opportunity to assume personal responsibility for their health. Many of the leading causes of death for people between the ages of 25 and 65 are preventable, wholly or in part, through changes in lifestyle. Not only can adults change established lifestyles, social norms related to health can be changed as well.

Behavioral changes have saved many adult lives in the past two decades. For example, the declines, by more than 40 percent and 50 percent, respectively, in coronary heart disease and stroke death rates since 1970, are associated with reduced rates of cigarette smoking, lower mean blood cholesterol, and increased control of high blood pressure. In the same period, deaths from motor vehicle crashes declined by almost 30 percent. Lower rates of alcohol use, increased seatbelt use, and changes in speed limits contributed to this reduction. Accompanying these trends were reduced public acceptance of certain risks, such as smoking and drinking and driving.

As deaths from heart disease have declined, cancer has became the leading cause of death for people aged 25 through 64 (Fig. 2.4). These and the other top causes of death between the ages of 25 and 65—unintentional injuries, stroke, and chronic liver disease and cirrhosis—have all been associated with risk factors related to lifestyle.

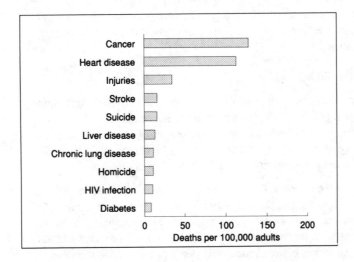

Fig. 2.4

Leading causes of death of adults aged 25 through 64 (1987)

Source: National Center for Health Statistics (CDC)

Cancer

Cancer, which is actually not one but many diseases, is associated with a variety of risk factors. Although cancer mortality rates overall have changed little since 1950, there have been significant changes in mortality for some age groups and cancers. Several prevalent forms of cancer can be either prevented or diagnosed early enough to prevent spread to other organs. It is estimated that 30 percent of cancer deaths are linked to smoking and that another large proportion, perhaps 35 percent, may be associated with diet.[19]

- **Lung cancer** is the most common—and most preventable—cancer in the United States for both men and women, and is increasing as large numbers of smokers grow older. Smoking is responsible for more than 85 percent of all lung cancer deaths. Since 1975, lung cancer incidence has risen more than 15 percent for black men, about 12 percent for black women, 12 percent for white men, and 8 percent for white women.[57]

- **Colorectal cancer** is the second leading cause of death due to cancer. Some studies have suggested that high fat and/or low fiber diets increase the risk of colorectal cancer. Since 1969, death rates from these cancers have fallen among white men and women, remained about the same for black women, and increased markedly for black men.[36] Although there is no general agreement that screening for colon cancer definitely reduces mortality among those not at high risk, consensus recommendations have suggested screening by digital rectal exams, fecal occult blood testing, and sigmoidoscopy for those over age 50.

- **Breast cancer** has become the second most common cause of cancer deaths among women, having been surpassed by lung cancer in the past decade. However, the incidence of breast cancer is more than twice that of lung cancer in women.[3] Early diagnosis of breast cancer improves the chance of survival significantly, with 90 percent of those diagnosed when the cancer was localized reaching the 5-year survival mark.[67] Breast cancer death rates could be reduced 30 percent with regular screening. Some evidence suggests that high-fat diets may increase the risk of breast cancer.

- **Cervical cancer** can be cured if detected early. Increased use of the Pap test has contributed to a 50-percent drop in cervical cancer deaths among both black and white women since 1969. However, black women continue to have 3 times the cervical cancer death rate of white women. Although the death rates have been decreasing, the *in situ* rates have risen in younger women aged 15 through 19.[3]

- **Oropharyngeal cancer**—cancer of the mouth and throat—accounts for 13.2 per 100,000 in 1987. Increased risk has been linked both to use of tobacco products and to heavy alcohol use.[70]

Heart Disease and Stroke

Despite a recent decline, coronary heart disease still kills more than 500,000 Americans annually. Another 1,250,000 people suffer nonfatal heart attacks each year.[46] About 20 percent of those who die from heart attacks are between the ages of 25 and 65, and most are between 55 and 64.[38] Quitting smoking, reducing dietary fat (especially saturated fat), and controlling high blood pressure can reduce the risk of heart disease.

Approximately 13 percent of the nearly 150,000 Americans who died of stroke in 1986 were between the ages of 25 and 64, and the majority of these were aged 55 through 64. Black men have the highest rate of stroke among all population groups, with a death rate from stroke about twice that of white men and a substantially higher rate than for black women. A much smaller gap exists between the stroke death rates of white men and white women.[38]

High blood pressure is a well-defined risk factor for both heart disease and stroke among adults. Approximately half of all heart attack victims and two-thirds of all stroke victims have high blood pressure.[46] About 30 percent of adults have high blood pressure (over 140/90 mm Hg or taking high blood pressure medication), but most do not have it under control.[43] It is estimated that, during 1982-84, only about 24 percent of hypertensive adults between 20 and 75 had achieved blood pressure control for 2 or more years.[46] Weight control, physical activity, lower intake of alcohol and sodium, and if necessary, medication are means of controlling blood pressure.[45]

Health Habits

Several major health risk factors, sometimes alone and sometimes in combination, are associated with the 5 major causes of death in the United States: cancer, heart disease, stroke, injury, and chronic lung disease. Reducing these risks has already significantly reduced the number of years of life lost before age 65, and greater reductions are possible.

Certain eating patterns—especially excessive consumption of fats—are linked to a higher risk of heart disease, breast and colon cancer, and gallbladder disease.[63] Total dietary fat, including saturated and unsaturated fats, now accounts for more than 36 percent of the total calories consumed in the United States. A fat intake of no more than 30 percent of calories is recommended by most groups, including the American Heart Association, the American Cancer Society, and the United States Departments of Agriculture and Health and Human Services.[63] These groups recommend that the major reduction in dietary fat come from saturated fats, which are common in foods from animal sources, such as meats and dairy products.

Overweight is a problem for about one-quarter of American adults, affecting about 27 percent of women and 24 percent of men.[41] This problem is associated with high blood pressure, elevated blood cholesterol, diabetes, heart disease, stroke, some cancers, and gall bladder disease. It also may be a factor in osteoarthritis of the weight-bearing joints.

Socioeconomic status has been linked to overweight. One national survey found that 37 percent of women below the poverty level were overweight, compared with 25 percent of those above the poverty level. Overweight is especially prevalent among members of some minority groups.[41]

To reduce this risk factor, both exercise and diet are important. As of 1985, however, only about 25 percent of overweight men and 30 percent of overweight women, among people 18 and over, were combining regular physical activity with sound dietary practices to lose weight.[66] Fewer than half of adult Americans exercise regularly (3 or more days a week, sustained for at least 20 minutes each time regardless of intensity)[7], a matter of concern because a sedentary lifestyle appears to be an independent risk factor for coronary heart disease. Older adults are less likely to be physically active than younger adults. Research increasingly suggests that even moderate physical activity can decrease the risk of coronary heart disease, especially among the sedentary. Regular physical activity can also help to prevent and manage hypertension, diabetes, osteoporosis, and obesity.[10] Further, it may play a role in mental health, having a favorable effect on mood, depression, anxiety, and self-esteem.

Cigarette smoking is an important risk factor for heart disease, stroke, and some forms of cancer. In 1965, 40 percent of all Americans smoked cigarettes. Today, that figure is below 30 percent. This dramatic decline is credited with saving nearly 800,000 lives between 1964 and 1985, with an average gain in life expectancy of 21 years for each death avoided or postponed. Despite these gains, smoking is still responsible for one of every six deaths in the United States. Moreover, it is still placing certain groups at greater risk of disease than others, and it is still the single most important preventable cause of death in our society.[57]

More than 50 million Americans still smoke. In 1987, 29 percent of adults aged 20 years and older smoked cigarettes. Almost as many have quit. By 1987, nearly half of those who ever smoked cigarettes (45 percent) had stopped. Since 1974, the rate of change for quitting has been similar for blacks and whites and for men and women.[60] Though more men smoke than women, the gender gap is decreasing. Prevalence of cigarette smoking has declined sharply among men since 1965 (from 50 to 32 percent) but only slightly among women (32 to 27 percent). In general, smoking rates are higher among blacks, Hispanics, blue-collar workers, and people with fewer years of education.[22]

Alcohol is a major factor in thousands of preventable deaths, including motor vehicle fatalities, homicides and suicides, cirrhosis of the liver, and some cancers, such as esophageal and liver cancer. Alcohol is also the leading preventable cause of birth defects.

There is evidence that the use of alcohol is beginning to decline. Based on alcoholic beverage sales and tax data, the consumption of hard liquor declined 21 percent between 1978 and 1986. Wine sales increased and beer sales remained about the same. While the overall trend in the consumption of alcoholic beverages is down, it is estimated that about 9 percent of people aged 21 and older consume more than two drinks daily.[50]

Increasing public concern about alcohol and other drugs, evident in many opinion polls, has helped galvanize organized action on the part of parent groups, government agencies, community groups, schools, and businesses.[6] Drinking and driving has been the focus of much of the attention: the Surgeon General has called for stricter regulation of advertising for alcoholic beverages; citizen groups have lobbied for and legislators have passed laws raising the drinking age and establishing stiff penalties for driving while intoxicated; the news media have devoted much coverage to the problem, and even the entertainment media have incorporated messages about drinking and driving into television programs.[56]

This widespread public concern and the programs that accompany it have had an impact. The proportion of motor vehicle deaths related to alcohol dropped by 10 to 15 percent between 1982 and 1986.[38] More recently, however, the decline has slowed, indicating the need for continued efforts.

Hospital emergency room visits related to use of illicit drugs, one indication of the health impact of drug abuse, rose sharply in the 1980s, and this high rate is expected to continue for some years. Cocaine is responsible for many of these visits. In 1987, cocaine-related emergency room visits constituted 32 percent of all visits related to drugs.[20] Other data indicate that young men between the ages of 25 and 44 are at a higher risk than the total population of being killed or injured by illicit drugs. In addition, drugs are implicated in about 10 percent of all homicides, many of which occur in this age group.

Seatbelt use is an important health habit, saving an estimated 4,000 lives in 1987, a year in which only about 42 percent of motor vehicle passengers used their seatbelts. Most of the crashes in which lives were saved by seatbelts occurred in States with mandatory seatbelt laws.[39] Passage of such laws in other States should increase usage and save many more lives. In addition, beginning with 1990 models, automobile manufacturers are equipping all passenger vehicles with automatic crash protection—automatic belts or airbags—in response to a new Federal requirement. Automatic belts are expected to increase overall usage to about 85 percent.[39]

Health Services

Preventing chronic disease depends often on individual decisions—to quit smoking, to drink in moderation if at all, to consume less saturated fat, to increase physical activity. What then is the role of health services?

One answer is patient education and counseling. Clinical studies have demonstrated that counseling by health professionals is effective in helping people change dietary and smoking behaviors. The U.S. Preventive Services Task Force, in surveying the effectiveness of 169 clinical interventions to prevent disease, concluded that counseling may be even more valuable overall than conventional clinical activities to prevent disease, such as many screening tests.[74]

Screening can be extremely important, when tailored appropriately to an individual's age and risk. Early diagnosis of disease can have a significant impact on mortality rates, as shown by the results of screening for high blood pressure and high blood cholesterol. The means are also available to detect various cancers when they are still curable, such as the Pap test for cervical cancer, mammography and physical examination for breast cancer, fecal occult blood testing and sigmoidoscopy for colorectal cancer, and skin examination for skin cancer. In 1987, just 75 percent of women aged 18 and over had received a

Pap test in the preceding one to three years, and this was by far the highest proportion of adults screened for any type of cancer.[37]

Only about 25 percent of women aged 50 and older surveyed in 1987, had received a mammogram and clinical breast exam in the preceding two years. The percentage of adults aged 50 and older who received a digital rectal exam and fecal occult blood testing in the preceding two years was estimated at 27 percent.[37]

Increasing awareness about preventive services by both health professionals and the public is essential to increasing their use. More and better insurance coverage for screening and counseling would also encourage wider use of these services. Expansion of managed care systems such as health maintenance organizations (HMOs) and preferred provider organizations (PPOs) can also provide basic preventive services to more people.

The challenge facing adults as individuals is to modify their lifestyles to maintain health and prevent disease. But even in adulthood, individual decisions are subject to many forces. Lifestyles once established are difficult to change, addictions even more difficult. Resolution of many of these difficulties is compounded by factors beyond the control of individuals. Socioeconomic status, the environment, community norms, media images and coverage, advertising, worksite standards, access to health care and counseling are powerful influences on adult behavior. So the other challenge facing adults, as members of society, is to work together to create an environment that facilitates and supports healthful behavior.

Many sectors of society have made a beginning. Some employers support smoking cessation, stress management, nutrition and exercise, screening for high blood pressure and high blood cholesterol, and other health-related programs. Hospitals provide patient education services and community health promotion programs. Community groups and churches sponsor classes and support groups. State agencies have initiated community-based prevention programs in many areas. In particular, minority communities, rural communities, and people with low incomes need relevant information and programs that address their particular risks and their need for preventive services.

Older Adults

In 1900, people over 65 constituted 4 percent of the population. By 1988, that proportion was up to 12.4 percent, by 2000 it will be 13 percent and by 2030, 22 percent. The most rapid population increase over the next decade will be among those over 85 years of age.[28]

People who reach the age of 65 can now expect to live into their eighties.[38] However, it is likely that not all those years will be active and independent ones. Thus, improving the functional independence, not just the length, of later life is an important element in promoting the health of this age group.

One measure of health that considers quality as well as length of life is the years of healthy life. While people aged 65 and older have 16.4 years of life remaining on average, they have about 12 years of healthy life remaining[21,38] (Fig. 2.5). Another indicator of quality of life is an individual's ability to perform activities required for daily living, such as bathing, dressing, and eating. Difficulty in performing these necessary tasks leads to the need for assistance and often limits opportunity for remaining independent in the community. People aged 85 and older constitute a substantial share of all people who are not independent in physical functioning.

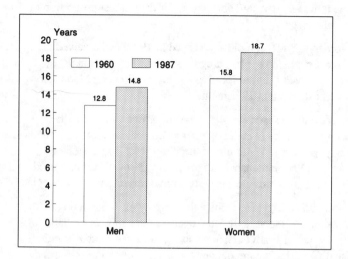

Fig. 2.5

Life expectancy at
age 65 by gender

Source: *Health, United
States, 1989 and Preven-
tion Profile*

While many people think of health problems in old age as inevitable, a substantial number are either preventable or can be controlled. The major causes of death among people aged 65 and older are heart disease, cancer, stroke, chronic obstructive pulmonary disease, pneumonia, and influenza. Chronic problems, such as arthritis, osteoporosis, incontinence, visual and hearing impairments, and dementia, are of equal concern because of their significant impact on day-to-day living. To accommodate the changing needs of an increasingly older society, we must prevent the ill from being disabled and help people with disabilities preserve function and prevent further disability.[26]

A growing body of evidence shows that changing certain health behaviors, even in old age, can benefit health and quality of life. Cigarette smoking is one of these habits. Studies have shown that when older smokers quit, they increase their life expectancy, reduce their risk of heart disease, and improve respiratory function and circulation.[57] Good nutrition is also important in the promotion and maintenance of health for older adults. Diet can play an important role in mitigating existing health problems with older people. Reducing sodium intake and losing weight, for example, can help keep blood pressure under control, and there is growing evidence that nutrition counseling and food programs can reduce the risk of disease among older adults.[28]

Physical Activity

A key ingredient to healthy aging is physical activity. Often physiological decline associated with aging may actually be the result of inactivity. Over 40 percent of people over age 65 report no leisure time physical activity.[7] Less than a third participate in regular moderate physical activity, such as walking and gardening, on a regular basis, and less than 10 percent engage routinely in vigorous physical activity. Yet regular physical activity and exercise are critical elements of health promotion for older adults. Increased levels of physical activity are associated with a reduced incidence of coronary heart disease, hypertension, noninsulin-dependent diabetes mellitus, colon cancer, and depression and anxiety which are diseases prominent in older adult populations.[10]

Moreover, increased physical activity increases bone mineral content, reduces the risk for osteoporotic fractures, helps maintain appropriate body weight, and increases longevity. It may also be that increased physical activity levels can improve balance, coordination, and strength, factors that may reduce the likelihood of falls in the older adult. Recent studies of exercise training among this age group have shown that older persons can adapt to increased levels of exercise with positive health benefits resulting from both high and low intensity exercise. In addition to these health benefits, a more important result of regular physical activity appears to be the maintenance of functional independence throughout the later years of life.

Health Services

People over age 65 need regular primary health care services to help them maintain their health and prevent disabling and life-threatening diseases and conditions. Clinical preventive services include the control of high blood pressure, screening for cancers, immunization against pneumonia and influenza, counseling to promote healthy behaviors, and therapies to help manage chronic conditions such as arthritis, osteoporosis, and incontinence. For example, skin cancer screening can detect the majority of malignant melanomas and basal cell carcinomas.

Especially important among these clinical services are those to detect breast cancer: screening mammography and clinical breast examination. These screening interventions are estimated to reduce mortality from breast cancer in women over age 50 by about 30 percent.[67] In addition, Pap tests to detect cervical cancer are important for older as well as for younger women.

Because pneumococcal disease is 3 times more prevalent among those over 65 than among younger people and takes many older lives, immunization of older adults is an important preventive service. Pneumonia was responsible for an average 48 days of restricted activity per 100 people aged 65 and older in 1987.[42] Likewise, immunization against influenza is recognized now as a basic preventive intervention for older adults. During 6 flu epidemics from 1972 to 1982, the death rate was 34 to 104 times higher in this age group than in younger people. Only about 10 percent of older adults living in the community receive pneumococcal vaccine and 20 percent receive influenza vaccines.[13]

The number of medicines prescribed to persons over the age of 65 increases the risk of adverse drug reactions, drug interactions, and other health problems associated with the use and misuse of medications. The risk of adverse reactions may be exacerbated by the physiological changes associated with aging. For example, decreased kidney and liver function can change the way the body processes medications. In some cases, the adverse effects of medication can be prevented by using a different drug or lower dose. Physicians, nurses, pharmacists and other health professionals can help reduce this risk through careful reviews of medication use and patient counseling.

Primary health care providers are necessary partners in the maintenance of good health and functional independence for older adults. In addition to ensuring appropriate screening, counseling, and immunization, they can monitor health status to detect early signs of other health problems that can threaten independence such as dementia or depression, as well as ensure an accurate distinction between the two in diagnosis. Alzheimer's disease is the best known and leading cause of cognitive impairment in older adults, but there are other, more treatable forms of dementia, characterized by deterioration of memory, orientation, general intellect, specific cognitive capacities, and social functioning. The prevalence of dementia ranges from about 5 to 10 percent of people over age 65, to 20 to 40 percent of those who have reached age 80. While most cases are not treatable, 10 to 20 percent of them—those caused by drug toxicity, metabolic disorders, depression, or hyperthyroidism—may be reversible.[16,34]

Providers can play an important role in identifying patients at risk for conditions for which interventions may be appropriate, e.g., counseling women at high risk for osteoporosis about the benefits and risks of estrogen replacement therapy. Urinary incontinence is another condition that can have serious consequences for functional independence. It affects many noninstitutionalized older adults and about half of all nursing home residents.[52] The risk of incontinence increases with age but it often is a sign of other problems. Various treatments are available, including pelvic muscle exercises and other behavioral treatments, drug therapy, and surgery. A major impediment is that only about half the people with incontinence report it to their physicians. Increased awareness of available treatments could reduce this often incapacitating problem.

Social Networks

Social isolation is both a risk factor for disease and a measure of reduced functional independence. Social support networks are of critical importance in promoting the health and independence of older adults.[28] Life changes common to the seventh and eighth decades can increase the risk of social isolation. Retirement and changes in social roles can affect systems of contact and support, as can the loss of spouses and close friends.

Depression, a frequent outcome of such changes, is of particular concern among older adults because of its impact on functional independence and its importance as a risk factor for suicide. Men aged 65 through 74 have the highest suicide rate in the United States.[12] Depression is treatable but often goes unsuspected by families and undiagnosed by physicians, perhaps because it is often only one of several health problems besetting an older adult. However, primary care providers who recognize the clinical signs and risk factors for depression—bereavement, loneliness, and low self-esteem—can help reduce suicide among older adults. Illness and disrupted marital status have also been linked to suicide in this age group.

Community support networks that provide services to help older adults maintain independence are also critical interventions for reducing social isolation. Primary care providers can also play a critical role, not only in the identification of individuals at risk, but also by supplying information and referral to available services.

References

1 Agency for Toxic Substances and Disease Registry. *The Nature and Extent of Lead Poisoning in Children in the United States: A Report to Congress.* Washington, DC: U.S. Department of Health and Human Services, 1988.

2 The Alan Guttmacher Institute. *Teenage Pregnancy: The Problem that Hasn't Gone Away.* New York: the Institute, 1981.

3 American Cancer Society. *Cancer Facts and Figures - 1989.* New York: the Society, 1990.

4 American School Health Association.

5 American School Health Association, Association of the Advancement of Health Education and Society for Public Health Education. *National Adolescent Student Health Survey.* Oakland, CA: Third Party Press, 1989.

6 Bachman, J.G.; Johnston, L.D.; O'Malley, P.M.; and Humphrey, R.H. Explaining the recent decline in marijuana use: Differentiating effects of perceived risks, disapproval, and general lifestyle factors. *Journal of Health and Social Behavior* 29:92-112, 1988.

7 Behavioral Risk Factor Surveillance System, Centers for Disease Control, Public Health Service, U.S. Department of Health and Human Services, Atlanta, GA.

8 Boyd, J.H and Moscicki, E.K. Firearms and youth suicide. *American Journal of Public Health* 76:1240-1242, 1986.

9 Bureau of the Census. *Educational Attainment in the United States: March 1987 and 1986.* Current Population Report, Series P-20, No. 428. Washington, DC: U.S. Department of Commerce, 1988.

10 Caspersen, C.J. Physical activity epidemiology: Concepts, methods, and applications to exercise science. *Exercise and Sport Sciences Reviews* 17:423-473, 1989.

11 Centers for Disease Control. *Homicide Surveillance: High Risk Racial and Ethnic Groups, Blacks and Hispanics, 1970 to 1983.* Atlanta, GA: U.S. Department of Health and Human Services, 1986.

12 Centers for Disease Control. *Suicide Surveillance, 1970-1980.* Atlanta, GA: Center for Health Promotion and Education, 1985.

13 Center for Infectious Diseases and Center for Prevention Services, Centers for Disease Control, Public Health Service, U.S. Department of Health and Human Services, Atlanta, GA.

14 Chasnoff, I.J. Drug use in women: Establishing a standard of care. *Annals of New York Academy of Sciences* 562:208, 1989.

15 Chasnoff, I.J.; Landress, H.J.; and Barrett, M.E. The prevalence of illicit drug and alcohol use during pregnancy and discrepancies in mandatory reporting in Pinellas County, Florida. *New England Journal of Medicine* 322:1202-6, 1990.

16 Clarfield, A.M. The reversible dementias: Do they reverse? *Annals of Internal Medicine* 109:476-86, 1988.

17 Clayton, R.R. The delinquency and drug use relationship among adolescents: A critical review. In: Lettieri, D.J. and Ludford, J. eds. *Drug abuse and the American adolescent.* NIDA Research Monograph 31. Rockville, MD: U.S. Department of Health and Human Services, 1981.

18 Division of Adolescent and School Health, Center for Chronic Disease Prevention and Health Promotion, Centers for Disease Control, Public Health Service, U.S. Department of Health and Human Services, Atlanta, GA.

19 Doll, R. and Peto, R. The causes of cancer: Quantitative estimates of avoidable risks of cancer in the United States today. *Journal of the National Cancer Institute* 66:1191-1308, 1981.

20 Drug Abuse Warning Network, National Institute on Drug Abuse, Alcohol, Drug Abuse, and Mental Health Administration, Public Health Service, U.S. Department of Health and Human Services, Rockville, MD.

21 Erikson, P. Unpublished analysis of vital statistics and National Health Interview Survey data, 1990.

22 Fiore, M.C.; Novotny, T.E.; Pierce, J.P.; Hatziandreu, E.J.; Patel, K.M.; and Davis R.M. Trends in cigarette smoking in the United States: The changing influence of race and gender. *JAMA* 261:49-55, 1989.

23 Furstenberg, F.F., Jr. *Unplanned Parenthood: The Social Consequences of Teenage Childbearing.* New York: Free Press, 1976.

24 Hall, J.R. A decade of detectors: Measuring the effect. *Fire Journal* 79:37-43, 1985.

25 Hollinshead, W.H. et al. Statewide prevalence of illicit drug use by pregnant women - Rhode Island. *Morbidity and Mortality Weekly Report* 39(14):225-7, 1990.

26 Institute of Medicine. *Disability in America: A National Agenda for Prevention.* edited by Pope, A. and Tarloff, A. Washington DC: National Academy Press, in press.

27 Institute of Medicine. *Preventing Low Birthweight.* Washington, DC: National Academy Press, 1985.

28 Institute of Medicine. *The Second Fifty Years: Promoting Health and Preventing Disability.* Washington DC: National Academy Press, in press.

29 Jones, E.F. and Forrest, J.D. Contraceptive failure in the United States: Revised estimates from the 1982 National Survey of Family Growth. *Family Planning Perspectives* 21(3):103-9, 1989.

30 Keith, L.G.; McGregor, S.N.; and Sciarra, J.J. Drug abuse in pregnancy. In: Chasnoff, I.J. ed. *Drugs, Alcohol, Pregnancy and Parenting.* Hingham, MA: Kluwer Academic Publishers, 1988.

31 Kleinman, J.C. and Kessel, S.S. Racial differences in low birthweight: trends and risk factors, *New England Journal of Medicine* 317:749-753, 1987.

32 Kleinman, J.C. and Kopstein, A. Smoking during pregnancy, 1967-1980. *American Journal of Public Health* 77:823-25, 1987.

33 Kleinman, J.C. and Madans, J.H. The effects of maternal smoking, physical stature, and educational attainment on the incidence of low birth weight. *American Journal of Epidemiology* 121(6):832-55, 1985.

34 Larson, E.B.; Reifler, B.V.; Featherstone, H.J.; et al. Dementia in elderly outpatients: A prospective study. *Annals of Internal Medicine* 100:417-23, 1984.

35 Mecham, P.J. et al. Suicide attempts among young adults. Paper presented at the 39th Annual Epidemic Intelligence Service Conference, Atlanta, GA. 1990.

36 National Cancer Institute. *1987 Annual Cancer Statistics Review.* DHHS Pub. No. (NIH)88-2789. Bethesda, MD: U.S. Department of Health and Human Services, 1988.

37 National Cancer Institute and the National Center for Health Statistics. Unpublished data from the Cancer Control Supplement to the 1987 National Health Interview Survey.

38 National Center for Health Statistics. *Health, United States, 1989 and Prevention Profile.* DHHS Pub. No. (PHS)90-1232. Hyattsville, MD: U.S. Department of Health and Human Services, 1990.

39 National Center for Statistics and Analysis. *Occupant Protection Facts.* Washington, DC: U.S. Department of Transportation, 1989.

40 National Commission to Prevent Infant Mortality. *Indirect Costs of Infant Mortality and Low Birthweight.* Washington, D.C: the Commission, 1988.

41 National Health and Nutrition Examination Survey (NHANES), National Center for Health Statistics, Centers for Disease Control, Public Health Service, U.S. Department of Health and Human Services, Hyattsville, MD.

42 National Health Interview Survey, National Center for Health Statistics, Centers for Disease Control, Public Health Service, U.S. Department of Health and Human Services, Hyattsville, MD.

43 National Heart, Lung, and Blood Institute. Hypertension prevalence and the status of awareness, treatment, and control in the U.S.: Final report of the subcommittee on definition and prevalence of the 1984 joint national committee. *Hypertension* 7(3): 457-468, 1985.

44 National Heart, Lung, and Blood Institute. *Report of the Expert Panel on Detection, Evaluation, and Treatment of High Blood Cholesterol in Adults.* National Cholesterol Education Program. Washington, DC: U.S. Department of Health and Human Services, 1988.

45 National Heart, Lung, and Blood Institute. *The 1988 Report of the Joint National Committee on Detection, Evaluation, and Treatment of High Blood Pressure.* Washington, DC: U.S. Department of Health and Human Services, 1988.

46 National Heart, Lung, and Blood Institute, National Institutes of Health, Public Health Service, U.S. Department of Health and Human Services, Bethesda, MD.

47 National Highway Traffic Safety Administration. *Fatal Accident Reporting System, 1987.* Washington, DC: U.S. Department of Transportation, 1988.

48 National Highway Traffic Safety Administration's 19 Cities Survey, U.S Department of Transportation, Washington, DC.

49 National Institute on Drug Abuse, Monitoring the Future Study (High School Senior Survey); Alcohol, Drug Abuse, and Mental Health Administration, Public Health Service, U.S. Department of Health and Human Services, Rockville, MD.

50 National Institute on Drug Abuse. *National Household Survey on Drug Abuse: Population Estimates, 1988.* DHHS Pub. No. (ADM)89-1636. Washington, DC: U.S. Department of Health and Human Services, 1989.

51 National Institute on Drug Abuse. *National Survey Results from High School, College, and Young Adult Populations, 1975-1988.* DHHS Pub. No. (ADM)89-1638. Washington, DC: U.S. Department of Health and Human Services, 1989.

52 National Institute of Health. Consensus Development Conference Statement: Urinary Incontinence in Adults, October 3-5, 1988.

53 National Research Council. *Risking the Future: Adolescent Sexuality, Pregnancy, and Childbearing.* Washington, DC: National Academy Press, 1987.

54 National School Boards Association. *Smoke-free Schools: A Progress Report.* Alexandria, VA: the Association, 1989.

55 National Survey of Family Growth. National Center for Health Statistics, Centers for Disease Control, Public Health Service, U.S. Department of Health and Human Services, Hyattsville, MD.

56 Office of Disease Prevention and Health Promotion. *Mass Communications and Health.* Washington, DC: U.S. Department of Health and Human Services, 1990.

57 Office on Smoking and Health. *Reducing the Health Consequences of Smoking: 25 Years of Progress. A Report of the Surgeon General.* DHHS Publication No. (CDC)89-8411. Washington, DC: U.S. Department of Health and Human Services, 1989.

58 Office of Technology Assessment. *Healthy Children: Investing in the Future.* Washington, DC: U.S. Congress, 1988.

59 Pamuk, E.R. and Mosher, W.D. Health aspects of pregnancy and childbirth: United States, 1982. In: *Vital and Health Statistics.* Series 23, No. 16. Hyattsville, MD: U.S. Department of Health and Human Services, 1988.

60 Pierce, J.P.; Fiore, M.C.; Novotny, T.E.; Hatziandreu, E.J.; and Davis, R.M. Trends in cigarette smoking in the United States: Projections to the year 2000 *JAMA* 261:61-65, 1989.

61 Pirie, P.L.; Murray, D.M.; and Luepker, R.V. Smoking prevalence in a cohort of adolescents, including absentees, drop outs, and transfers. *American Journal of Public Health* 78:176-78, 1988.

62 President's Committee on Mental Retardation. *Preventing the New Morbidity: A Guide for State Planning for the Prevention of Mental Retardation and Related Disabilities Associated with Socioeconomic Conditions.* Washington, DC: U.S. Deaprtment of Health and Human Services, 1988.

63 Public Health Service. *The Surgeon General's Report on Nutrition and Health.* Washington, DC: U.S. Department of Health and Human Services, 1988.

64 *Report to Congress and the White House on the Nature and Effectiveness of Federal, State, and Local Drug Prevention/Education Programs.* Washington, DC: U.S. Department of Education, 1987.

65 Rouse, B.A. Epidemiology of smokeless tobacco use: national study. *NCI Monograph* 8:29-33, 1989.

66 Schoenborn, C.A. Health promotion and disease prevention: United States, 1985. *Vital and Health Statistics,* Series 10, No. 163. DHHS Pub. No. (PHS)88-1591, Hyattsville, MD: U.S. Department of Health and Human Services, 1988.

67 Shapiro, S.; Venet, W.; Strax, L.; and Roeser, R. Selection, follow-up, and analysis in the Health Insurance Plan Study: A randomized trial with breast cancer screening. *NCI Monographs* 67:65-74, 1985.

68 Shapiro S.; McCormick, M.C.; Starfield, B.H.; Krischer, J.P.; and Bross, D. Relevance of correlates of infant deaths for significant morbidity at one year of age. *American Journal of Obstetrics and Gynecology* 136:363-373, 1980.

69 Sonnenstein, F.L.; Pleck, J.H.; and Ku, L.C. Sexual activity, condom use, and AIDS awareness among adolescent males. *Family Planning Perspectives* 21(4):152-8, 1989.

70 Surveillance, Epidemiology, and End Results (SEER) Program, National Cancer Institute, National Institutes of Health, Bethesda, MD.

71 Taffel, S.M. Maternal weight gain and the outcome of pregnancy. *Vital and Health Statistics,* Series 21, No. 44, DHHS Pub. No. (PHS)86-1922. Washington, DC: U.S. Department of Health and Human Services, 1986.

72 U.S. Department of Health and Human Services. National children and youth fitness study II. *Journal of Physical Education, Recreation, and Dance* 58:50-96, 1987.

73 U.S. Department of Health and Human Services. *Report of the Secretary's Task Force on Black and Minority Health.* Washington, DC: the Department, 1985.

74 U.S. Preventive Services Task Force. *Guide to Clinical Preventive Services: An Assessment of the Effectiveness of 169 Interventions.* Baltimore, MD: Williams and Wilkins, 1989.

75 Westat, Inc. *Study Findings: Study of National Incidence of Child Abuse and Neglect.* Washington, DC: U.S. Department of Health and Human Services, 1988.

3. The Nation's Health: Special Populations

Progress toward a healthier America will depend substantially on improvements for certain populations that are at especially high risk. For that reason, *Healthy People 2000* sets specific targets to narrow the gap between the total population and those population groups that now experience above average incidences of death, disease, and disability. These population groups include people with low incomes, people who are members of some racial and ethnic minority groups, and people with disabilities. Likewise, it sets specific targets for controlling some of the risk factors that contribute to the disease burden of groups at highest risk. Special population groups often need targeted preventive efforts, and such efforts require understanding the needs and the particular disparities experienced by these groups. General solutions cannot always be used to solve specific problems.

This section provides profiles of the at-risk population groups addressed by *Healthy People 2000*: low-income groups, minority groups, and people with disabilities. At the outset, it is necessary to point to two caveats that limit these profiles and pose major health challenges in themselves.

First, data are limited; sometimes, and for some groups, the data may be severely limited. Without data, targets cannot be set, even though professional consensus exists that a population group is at considerably higher risk than the total population. A challenge of the coming years is to build better data systems, at national and State levels, in order that the scope of health threats facing various groups within our society can be adequately defined and appropriate preventive interventions can be effectively focused.

Second, the special populations themselves are extremely heterogenous. Whether the group is defined as low income, black, Hispanic, Asian and Pacific Islander Americans, American Indians and Alaska Natives, or people with disabilities, the variations within each group are extensive. Generalizations, which characterize population profiles by definition, are dangerous because the exceptions are many. The challenge is to refine our knowledge and our understanding even further, especially as basic health policies are translated into community-based prevention programs and clinical preventive services.

With these two caveats in mind, profiles of special populations can be used, together with those in the preceding section that address age groups, to provide the human context for the health strategy laid out in this report.

People with Low Income

Nearly 1 of every 8 Americans lives in a family with an income below the Federal poverty level. Nearly a quarter of children younger than 6 are members of such families.[11] Low income itself (or low socioeconomic status) is a shorthand label that encompasses family groups with individuals who have poorly paid jobs or are unemployed, families living in substandard housing, and families more likely to have only a single parent in residence. Health disparities between poor people and those with higher incomes are almost universal for all dimensions of health. Those disparities may be summarized by the finding that people with low income have death rates that are twice the rates for people with incomes above the poverty level.[1]

For virtually all of the chronic diseases that lead the Nation's list of killers, low income is a special risk factor. For example, the risk of death from heart disease is more than 25 percent higher for low income people than for the overall population.[16] The incidence of cancer increases as family income decreases, and survival rates are lower for low-income cancer patients. The association of cancer and low income varies by cancer site; lung, esophageal, oral, stomach, cervical, and prostate cancers are more frequent among the poor, while breast and colorectal cancers are not.[1,30] Infectious diseases, like HIV infection and tuberculosis, are also often found disproportionately among the poor.

Similar vulnerability for low income people is found with some causes of traumatic injury and death. These individuals, more than those with higher incomes, are the victims of violent crime. Poverty appears to be a major predisposing factor associated with a higher risk for murder of acquaintances and family members, as well as robbery-motivated killings of strangers. Injuries and deaths among children from fires, drowning, and suffocation are strongly related to low socioeconomic status.[11]

No single indicator of health status makes the connection between poverty and poor health more clear than does infant mortality. Poor pregnancy outcomes including prematurity, low birth weight, birth defects, and infant death are linked to low income, low educational level, low occupational status, and other indicators of social and economic disadvantage.[8]

Poverty reduces a person's prospects for long life by increasing the chances of infant death, chronic disease, and traumatic death; poverty is also often associated with significant developmental limitations. For example, iron deficiency is more than twice as common in low income children, aged 1 and 2, as it is among the total population of that age.[14] Growth retardation affects 16 percent of low income children younger than age 6. In the mid-1980s, an estimated 3 million children, virtually all of them from low income families, had blood lead levels that exceeded 15 µg/dL, sufficient to place them at risk for impaired mental and physical development. The rate of mental retardation is reported to be higher among children in poverty. Poor children experience more sickness from infection and other debilitating conditions than the total population. Children in families with incomes below $5,000 per year had an average of 9.1 disability days in 1980 compared to only 4 days for children in families with incomes of $25,000 or more.[15]

The pattern of increased vulnerability to injury, disease, and death continues into adulthood. People in families with incomes of less than $13,000 a year are twice as likely as the total population to be limited in major activities because of their health (Fig. 3.1). Activity limitations are four times more common among people with 8 years or less of education than among those with 16 years or more. Bed disability days increase as income decreases.[17]

Just as poor health is more likely among persons of low income, so are some, but not all, of the major risk factors for poor health. Higher-than-average rates of obesity and high

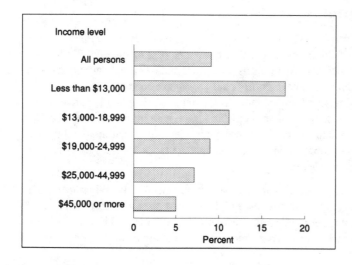

Fig. 3.1

Percentage of people who experience limitation of major activity, by income level (1988, age-adjusted)

Source: National Health Interview Survey (CDC)

blood pressure, which are major risks for heart disease and stroke, have been linked directly with low income status.[23] Tobacco use, which has declined dramatically in the past two decades for the population as a whole, has remained virtually constant since 1966 for those who completed less than 12 years of schooling. Smoking levels among blue-collar workers are about 20 percent higher than among others.[21]

Whereas in 1986 over 15 percent of people under age 65 had no health insurance either by private or public forms of coverage, lack of health insurance coverage was a problem for 37 percent of families with incomes below $10,000 a year.[12]

In 1987 only 22 percent of low-income women over age 40 had ever received a clinical breast examination and a mammogram, as compared to 36 percent of women in the total population.[15] Relatively low survival rates for breast cancer among low-income women point to the need for earlier diagnosis and treatment. While the benefits of prenatal care for low-income women are well documented, with a savings-cost ratio on the order of 3-to-1, low utilization rates are characteristic of groups at high risk of low birth weight and other maternal and infant health problems.[8] Approximately 40 percent of children from low-income families have untreated dental caries, another indicator of the lack of preventive and primary health care.[20]

For the coming decade, perhaps no challenge is more compelling than that of equity. The disparities experienced by people who are born and live their lives at the lowest income levels define the dimensions of that challenge. The relationships between poverty and health are complex and cannot be reduced to a simple one-to-one relationship between dollars available and level of health. Low income may, in fact, be a product of poor health, just as poor health may be caused by environmental exposures, material deficiencies, and lack of access to health services that adequate income might correct or improve. While, from a public health perspective, the leverage available to effect improvements is limited largely to the availability and the quality of health services, improvements in education, job training, and other social services are necessary to erase the health effects of current income disparities.

People in Minority Groups

The United States has been called a "melting pot" of ethnic and racial groups. In recent decades, it has become clearer that the image is no longer an appropriate one. Rather than amalgamating into one single group, we have come to recognize and even celebrate our diversity as a basis for national strength. Nevertheless, our health care programs are characterized by unacceptable disparities linked to membership in certain racial and ethnic groups.

The predominant minority populations of the United States can be categorized as blacks, Hispanics, Asian and Pacific Islander Americans, and American Indians and Alaska Natives. From a total population perspective, the categories simplify the difficulties of assessing health status and making plans to improve health. But they are gross simplifications. Within each racial or ethnic category, significant subgroup differences exist. Demarcations among minority populations are not absolute. For example, there are both black and nonblack Hispanics. Many nonblack Hispanics share historic roots and genetic endowments that are closely related to those of many American Indian groups, while others have European roots and do not share the genetic make-up which may predispose to adult-onset diabetes. Alaska Natives may have more in common with some Asians than they do with American Indians in the lower 48 States. In short, differences within the principal population groups must always temper generalizations about their health needs.

The extent of disparities suffered by minority groups in America was documented in the mid-1980s by the *Report of the Secretary's Task Force on Black and Minority Health*.[30] This report found that black Americans suffered nearly 60,000 excess deaths per year in the period 1979-1980, with "excess deaths" defined as the difference between the number of deaths observed in that minority population and the number of deaths that would have been expected if that population had the same age- and gender-specific death rate as the white population.

A compelling disparity of most minority populations in the United States is socio-economic. The discussion on low-income people describes a small portion of the white American population. It applies to much larger portions of those from black, Hispanic, Asian and Pacific Islander, and American Indian and Alaska Native communities. Poverty and near-poverty appear as underlying elements of many health problems experienced by these groups. But if the socioeconomic effects are set aside, disparities experienced by these population groups will still be observed. Simply put, some differences in survival and health are not solely explained by poverty or other environmental factors.[4] For that reason, *Healthy People 2000* assesses disparities not only in terms of income level and educational attainment, but also in terms of the Nation's racial and ethnic population groups. Special population targets for improvements to be achieved by 2000 are set for those groups with higher risks than the total population, where data are available to establish such targets.

Black Americans

African Americans make up 12 percent of the United States population, thereby constituting the Nation's largest minority group. Members of this group live in all regions of the country and are represented in every socioeconomic group. One-third of blacks live in poverty, a rate three times that of the white population. Over half live in central cities, in areas often typified by poverty, poor schools, crowded housing, unemployment, exposure to a pervasive drug culture and periodic street violence, and generally high levels of stress. Life expectancy for blacks has lagged behind that for the total population throughout this century; since the mid-1980s the gap has actually widened, with the life expectancy rising to 75 years for the overall population while falling slightly for blacks, from a high of 69.7 years in 1984 to 69.4 years in 1987.[3] The leading chronic diseases as causes of death for black Americans are the same as those for the majority population (Fig. 3.2). However, black men die from strokes at almost twice the rate of men in the total population, and their risk of nonfatal stroke is also higher. Coronary heart disease death rates do not show such disparate levels, although death rates are higher for black women than for white women. On the other hand, when heart disease rates are compared within income levels, black rates are lower than those for whites.[30]

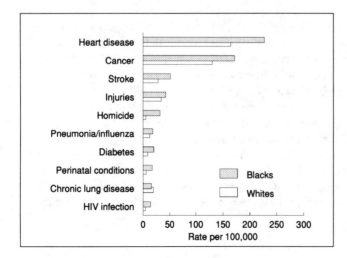

Fig. 3.2

Leading causes of death for blacks compared to whites (1987, age-adjusted rates)

Source: National Center for Health Statistics (CDC)

Black men also experience a higher risk of cancer than nonblack men, with a 25-percent higher risk of all cancers and a 45-percent higher incidence of lung cancer. Only 38 percent of blacks with cancer survive 5 years after diagnosis, compared to 50 percent of whites.[30]

Diabetes is 33 percent more common among blacks than whites. The highest rates are among black women, especially those who are overweight. The complications of diabetes—heart disease, stroke, kidney failure, and blindness—all are more prevalent among blacks with diabetes than whites with diabetes.[30]

Black babies are twice as likely as white babies to die before their first birthday. High rates of low birth weight among black babies account for many of these deaths, but even normal-weight black babies have a greater risk of death. Black infant mortality rates are higher not only for babies in the first month of life, but also for those between 1 month and 1 year of age. The major killer in this period is sudden infant death syndrome (SIDS). Other causes of death that are more prevalent for black infants than for the total population include respiratory distress syndrome, infections, and injuries.[19]

Homicide is the most frequent cause of death for black men between the ages of 15 and 34. The homicide rate for those between ages 25 and 34 is 7 times that of whites. A black man has a 1-in-21 lifetime chance of being murdered, and black women are more than four times as likely to be homicide victims as white women.[30] Most young black murder victims are killed with firearms in the course of an argument. It is estimated that about half of all homicides in the United States are related to alcohol use and 10 percent or more to the use of illegal drugs.

The rate of AIDS among blacks is more than triple that of whites. Among women and children, the gaps are even wider. Black women face between 10 and 15 times the risk of AIDS as compared to white women. Black children account for more than 50 percent of all children with AIDS. The proportion of AIDS cases associated with intravenous drug abuse is greater for blacks than for other AIDS victims, and higher rates of heterosexual transmission of the HIV virus and transmission of the virus from mother to infant occur as a consequence.[26]

Disparities in the experience of health risks mirror some of the most striking disparities in health outcomes. High blood pressure is much more common among blacks of both genders than among the total population. Severe high blood pressure is present 4 times more often among black men than among white men.[29] Overweight is a problem for 44 percent of black women aged 20 and older, compared to 37 percent for low income women and 27 percent for all women. Poor nutrition, smoking, alcohol and drug abuse, and other risk factors appear more commonly among blacks with low incomes.[30]

Adolescent pregnancy is a major concern among the black population, for its social and economic consequences as much as for its health effects. There are higher risks of infant mortality and low birth weight, especially for very young pregnant girls. But even greater risks indirectly threaten the health of both mother and baby because of the patterns of poverty and low educational attainment that often become solidified as a result of early childbearing. Actual rates of childbirth among black teenagers have dropped since the 1960s, but because the number of girls in this population has risen by 20 percent, the total number of births has increased. In 1987, births among girls aged 15 through 17 were 3 times as likely among black girls as among white girls. Birth rates among black girls younger than 15 were nearly 5 times higher, than the rate for white girls.[12]

Statistics demonstrate with sharp clarity that blacks do not receive enough early, routine, and preventive health care. Early prenatal care can reduce low birth weight and prevent infant deaths. Early detection of cancers can increase survival rates. Appropriate medical care can reduce the frequency and severity of the complications of diabetes, which

blacks experience at higher rates than others. Information about actual use of h   are
services confirm these indications. Blacks make fewer annual visits to physici   .n
whites, and black mothers are twice as likely as white mothers to receive no healu   are
or care only in the last trimester of their pregnancies.[30] Hospital emergency rooms and
clinics are a much more common source of medical care for blacks than for whites, and
20 percent of blacks compared to 13 percent of whites report no usual source of medical
care.[30] Though recent statistics are not available to assess immunization coverage by
race, children in central cities—many of whom are black Americans—lagged as much as
20 percent behind immunization rates for children living in other places. In 1986, about
23 percent of blacks had no private or public medical insurance, compared to 14 percent
of whites.[12]

Hispanic Americans

The Hispanic subgroups—Mexican Americans, Puerto Ricans, Cuban Americans,
Central and South American immigrants, and other Spanish-surname/Spanish-speaking
communities—compose the second largest minority group in the United States. At the
beginning of the 1990s, they constitute about 8 percent of the total population and are the
fastest growing minority group. Over 70 percent of Hispanics were born in this country.
Within the Hispanic populations, Mexican Americans are nearly two-thirds of the total,
Puerto Ricans (excluding those who live in Puerto Rico) are 12 percent, Cuban Americans are 5 percent, people of Central and South American origin are 11 percent, and
others (including Spanish-speaking immigrants from Caribbean islands) make up 9 percent. Eighty-seven percent of Hispanics live in urban areas. The largest concentrations
of Mexican Americans are in Western States, notably California and Texas. More Puerto
Ricans reside in East Coast States, led by New York. Cuban Americans more often
reside in Florida.[13]

Hispanics experience perhaps the most varied set of health issues facing a single minority
population. Whereas Mexican Americans have low rates of cerebrovascular disease,
stroke rates among New York Puerto Ricans are high. Cuban Americans have high
utilization rates for prenatal care, but lower rates prevail among Mexican Americans and
Puerto Ricans. Infant mortality rates vary substantially from group to group (Fig. 3.3).
In short, the Hispanic health profile is marked by diversity. This diversity is intertwined
with the ever-present effects of socioeconomic status, and with geographic and cultural
differences.

Two related demographic facts are especially important for the health issues and
prospects of the Hispanic population: its youthfulness and its high birth rate. The

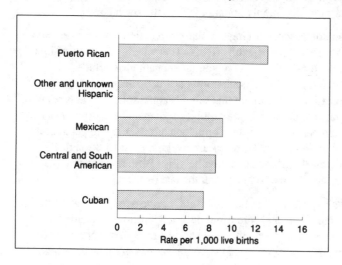

Fig. 3.3
Infant mortality rates
for selected Hispanic
groups (1983-84)

Source: National Linked
Birth and Infant Death
Data Set (CDC)

median Hispanic age is less than 26, compared to about 33 for the total population. Approximately 38 percent of all Hispanics are aged 19 and younger.[3] The Hispanic birth rate was 22.3 births per 1,000 women in 1987, while that of the total population was 15.7 births per 1,000 women.[19]

The leading causes of death among Hispanic Americans document several differences between their health experience and that of the total population (Fig. 3.4). Heart disease and cancer lead the list, as is the case for other Americans, but death rates from these 2 causes are actually lower than for non-Hispanics. Unintentional injuries, homicide, chronic liver disease and cirrhosis, and AIDS rank higher on the Hispanic list; suicide, stroke, and chronic obstructive pulmonary disease rank lower.[13] In the case of homicide, the great majority of victims are young men. In the southwest, Hispanic men aged 20 through 24 have 4 times the homicide rate of their non-Hispanic, white counterparts.[28] In the case of AIDS, Hispanics' rate is nearly 3 times higher than for non-Hispanic whites, with rates among Puerto Rican-born Hispanics as much as 7 times higher.[27] The cumulative incidence of AIDS among Hispanic women is about 8 times higher than among non-Hispanic women, and the rate for HIV infection over 6 times higher for Hispanic children. As with black Americans, HIV transmission among Hispanic women is primarily linked to intravenous drug abuse by these women or their sexual partners.[27] Diabetes is especially prevalent among Mexican Americans.[13]

Hispanics		*Rank*	*White non-Hispanics*	
Heart disease	25%	1	Heart disease	37%
Cancer	17%	2	Cancer	23%
Injuries	9%	3	Stroke	7%
Stroke	6%	4	Chronic lung disease	4%
Homicide	5%	5	Injuries	4%
Liver disease	3%	6	Pneumonia/ influenza	4%
Pneumonia/ influenza	3%	7	Diabetes	2%
Diabetes	3%	8	Suicide	2%
HIV infection	3%	9	Atherosclerosis	1%
Perinatal conditions	3%	10	Liver disease	1%

Fig. 3.4

Leading causes of death for Hispanics and white non-Hispanics in 18 States and the District of Columbia, as a percent of total deaths (1987)

Source: *Monthly Vital Statistics Report*, Supplement, September 26, 1989

Note: National death rate data unavailable for Hispanics.

Among the risks to health, smoking continues among 43 percent of Hispanic men, and Hispanic teenagers of both genders smoke more than do either non-Hispanic black or non-Hispanic white teenagers. Likewise, Hispanic teenagers report heavy drinking of alcoholic beverages more frequently than do white or black teenagers. Puerto Ricans and Cuban Americans aged 12 through 17 report higher rates of cocaine use than do either whites or blacks, and Mexican Americans have higher rates of marijuana use. Cocaine-related deaths tripled between 1982 and 1984 among Hispanics, while they were doubling among non-Hispanic whites.[13]

Overweight is common among Hispanics, especially among Mexican American women. This disparity cannot be accounted for completely by socioeconomic differences. Likewise, Mexican Americans participating in a San Antonio Heart Study were found to have physical activity rates lower than those in the total population, even after differences in socioeconomic status, residential location, and gender were taken into account.[13]

Like black Americans, Hispanic Americans receive less preventive health care, including prenatal care, than the total population. In 1987, 39 percent of Hispanic mothers had no prenatal care during the first trimester of pregnancy compared to 21 percent of non-Hispanic whites.[12] Barriers to care include language differences between Spanish-speaking patients and English-speaking health professionals, logistical barriers posed by rural residence of some Hispanic families, and costs of services.

Migrant farmworkers, a small but important subset of Hispanic Americans, deserve special attention. Migrant farmworkers may also belong to white, black, Haitian, or other ethnic groups, but the largest group is Hispanic. Their infant mortality rate is about 25 percent greater than that of the national average; their life expectancy is 49 years rather than 75 years; the rate of parasitic infection among some sets of farm workers approaches 50 times that of the total population.[18] The health care needs of these farmworkers are particularly challenging, given their migratory patterns, low incomes, poor education, and lack of health insurance.

Asian and Pacific Islander Americans

The diversity that characterizes the more than 11 million people who are Asian and Pacific Islanders is striking. As a whole, they are the Nation's third largest minority group, but this single label is an oversimplification. They speak over 30 different languages and bring with them a similar number of distinct cultures. Approximately three-quarters of them are immigrants, mostly from Southeast Asia, and many of them are refugees. A small proportion are either immigrants from South Pacific islands or Native Hawaiians.[3]

From the perspective of their health prospects, those born within the United States and established here for generations are virtually undistinguishable from the population as a whole. Indeed, their median income is higher than that of the overall United States population, with Japanese families having annual incomes 38-percent higher than the national median income. Yet, some groups, particularly recent immigrants, are extremely poor. For example, Laotian immigrants have one of the highest poverty rates of any group in the Nation. Even within subgroups, diversity characterizes both socioeconomic and health profiles. While Chinese Americans generally enjoy adequate incomes and relatively good health, communities such as Chinatown in San Francisco have higher poverty levels. Elimination of the disparities between Asian and Pacific Islander Americans and the general population may parallel integration of the newer immigrants into both the economy and the society of the United States.

An adequate depiction of the health of Asian and Pacific Islander Americans is constrained because data cannot be stratified by subgroups. Many national data systems are unable to make estimates of this minority population because of its relatively small size. This prevents accurate assessment of the leading causes of death, disease, and disability that it experiences. From local studies, however, it is possible to recognize certain diseases as posing higher than normal risks for specific Asian and Pacific Islander Americans. Most of the studies are based in California, which has the largest Asian and Pacific Islander American population (Fig. 3.5). Generalizations from local studies may be inaccurate and misleading due to the profound differences among Asian and Pacific Islander American groups, for example the difference in perinatal mortality among the groups (Fig. 3.6).

Disparities in rates of cancer exist for several subgroups and selected cancer sites. For example, the breast cancer incidence rate among Native Hawaiians is 111 per 100,000 women, as compared to 86 per 100,000 among whites.[2] The lung cancer rate is 18 percent higher among Southeast Asian men than for the white population. And the liver cancer rate is more than 12 times higher among Southeast Asians than in the white population.[2,25] Higher rates of high blood pressure have been found among Filipinos aged 50 and older living in California (61 percent for men and 65 percent for women) than among the total California population (47 percent).[30]

Asians and Pacific Islanders		Rank	Whites	
Heart disease	28%	1	Heart disease	35%
Cancer	24%	2	Cancer	23%
Stroke	9%	3	Stroke	8%
Injuries	7%	4	Chronic lung disease	5%
Pneumonia/ influenza	4%	5	Pnuemonia/ influenza	4%
Chronic lung disease	3%	6	Injuries	4%
Suicide	2%	7	Suicide	2%
Diabetes	2%	8	Liver disease	2%
Perinatal conditions	2%	9	Diabetes	1%
Liver disease	1%	10	Atherosclerosis	1%

Fig. 3.5

Leading causes of death for Asians and Pacific Islanders and whites in California, as a percent of total deaths (1987)

Source: California State Department of Health and Asian American Health Forum

Note: California's published data on the Asian and Pacific Islander population includes 93 percent Asians and 7 percent Other (Native Americans, Eskimos, and Alaskan Aleuts.) National death rate data are unavailable for Asians and Pacific Islanders.

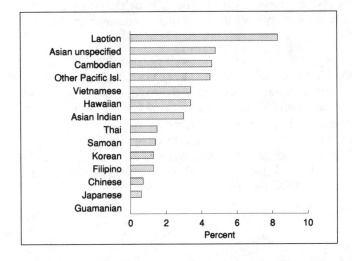

Fig. 3.6

Percent of deaths attributed to conditions originating in the perinatal period, for selected Asian groups

Source: California State Department of Health and Asian American Health Forum

The two infectious diseases that have followed immigrant Asian and Pacific Islander population subgroups to this country are tuberculosis and hepatitis B. Tuberculosis is still the leading cause of death in some Asian countries and has become a serious health problem in some Asian communities in large American cities. Among Southeast Asian immigrants, the incidence is 40 times higher than in the total population. Rates are particularly high among those over age 45.[2] Higher rates of hepatitis B are also found among Asian immigrants. This infection is associated with chronic liver disease, cirrhosis, and liver cancer. The overall carrier rate in the United States is estimated to be 0.3 percent of the population; among immigrants from Southeast Asia the estimated rate is 4 percent. Infection is spread from mother to infant and from child to child. Refugee transit camps now screen pregnant women and vaccinate infants of those who are carriers of hepatitis B and all children under age 6.[5] Among the risk factors of greatest concern is smoking. Among California immigrant groups, smoking rates among men are 92 percent for Laotians, 71 percent for Cambodians, and 65 percent for Vietnamese, compared to 30 percent for the overall American population.[2]

Faced with western medicine and a health care system that is unfamiliar, Americans of Asian and Pacific Island heritage experience unique access barriers to primary care. In addition to linguistic and cultural differences, financial problems beset many subgroups, especially recent immigrants and refugees.

American Indians and Alaska Natives

Descendants of the original residents of North America now number approximately 1.6 million and compose the smallest of the defined minority groups. Diversity characterizes this group, too, encompassing numerous tribes and over 400 federally recognized nations, each with its own traditions and cultural heritage. Eskimos, Aleuts, and Indians residing in Alaska are referred to as Alaska Natives; those residing in other States are referred to as American Indians. The Federal Government collects detailed data on American Indians and Alaska Natives in 33 States that include reservations; health care services are provided through the Indian Health Service to those living in these reservation States. Thus, it is possible to derive a composite profile of this population group. However, only about one-third of this group lives on reservations or historic trust lands, while about 50 percent live in urban centers.

In general, the American Indian and Alaska Native population is youthful. The median age of those living in the reservation States is about 23, compared to over 32 for the United States population as a whole. Income and educational levels tend to be low, with more than 1 in 4 living below the poverty level and fewer than 8 percent having college degrees.[6]

One reason for the youthfulness of the population is the large proportion of the population who die before age 45. Most of the excess deaths—those that would not have occurred if American Indian death rates were comparable to those of the total population—can be traced to 6 causes: unintentional injuries, cirrhosis, homicide, suicide, pneumonia, and complications of diabetes (Fig. 3.7). Heart disease and cancer are not among the sources of excess deaths, perhaps because these are generally diseases of older age. Cancer rates are lower overall, but are twice as high as the total population for lung cancer among Oklahoma Indians. Southwest Indians have high rates of gallbladder cancer, and Alaska Natives suffer high rates of liver cancer.[30]

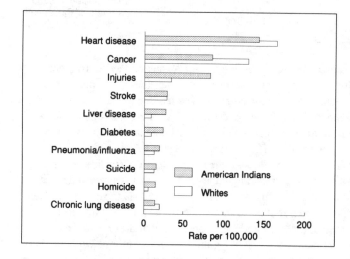

Fig. 3.7

Leading causes of death for American Indians in Reservation States compared to whites (1987, age-adjusted rates)

Source: Indian Health Service and National Center for Health Statistics (CDC)

The second leading cause of death among American Indian men, and the first cause for those younger than age 44, is unintentional injuries, accounting for over one-fifth of all their deaths each year.[19] An estimated 75 percent of these injuries are alcohol-related, and 54 percent involve motor vehicle crashes. Alcohol is also a factor in a homicide rate that is 60 percent higher than that of the total population. Suicide, the third of the four alcohol-related causes of death among American Indians, occurs at an overall rate that is

28 percent higher than the national rate, but among some tribes the suicide rate is 10 times higher than the total population rate.[6]

Cirrhosis and diabetes are the two chronic diseases that afflict American Indians more frequently than other groups. Cirrhosis deaths occur at about three times the total population rate, and cirrhosis is the fourth alcohol-related health effect contributing significantly to death and disability among American Indians.[24] Diabetes is now so prevalent that in many tribes more than 20 percent of the members have this disease.[6] Among two tribes in Arizona, the rate is 40 percent of adults. Obesity contributes to the high incidence of diabetes experienced by many American Indian communities, and it is also linked to hypertension and cardiovascular disease. The increase in obesity among American Indians in the last 50 years has paralleled the increasing rates of diabetes.

Alcohol and obesity are risk factors that stand out as problems for the American Indian population. One estimate is that 95 percent of American Indian families are affected either directly or indirectly by a family member's alcohol abuse.[24] While American Indians living on reservations and tribal members with access to reservation health facilities are served by the Indian Health Service, access to health care is still a problem for many. Many live in rural areas where the availability of physicians is about half that of the national average and where the Indian Health Service may not provide health care services. Health problems may appear especially intractable, but gains achieved among a number of tribes in reducing infant mortality rates to levels below those of the population as a whole provide testimony to the possibility of major improvement in the coming decade.

People With Disabilities

Throughout this document, the preventive actions implicit in targets to be achieved by 2000 seek not only to reduce unnecessary deaths and the immediate suffering and costs of infectious and chronic diseases; they also seek to prevent the longer-term consequences of functional impairments that can severely affect the quality of one's life. As a prevention plan for the 1990s, *Healthy People 2000* addresses not only the prevention of premature death and disease, but also the prevention of disabilities. Even when data are unavailable to define health outcomes except in terms of death, the thrust of objectives for the year 2000 is aimed at the living consequences of unhealthy behaviors, unsafe environments, and illness-causing infections. Disabilities may be defined, as distinct from illness or disease, in terms of limited ability to function. Disabilities may be physical or mental; and they may include motor or sensory limitations. The focus is on effects, rather than causes, since a similar functional limitation, such as a limitation in ability to walk, may be caused by a congenital birth defect, an injury, or a leg amputation resulting from complications of diabetes.

When the focus is on prevention of disabilities, another group of Americans who face special health risks becomes evident: those who already experience serious and chronic disability. The health promotion and disease prevention needs of people with disabilities are not nullified because they were born with an impairing condition or have experienced a disease or injury that has long-term consequences. In fact, those needs for health promotion are accentuated. People with disabilities are at higher risk of future problems that can only increase the limitations that they experience. For that reason, *Healthy People 2000* addresses people with disabilities as a special population, and where data are available, sets specific targets to address their needs and enhance their health.

Secondary conditions—health problems that arise from, or are related to, the main cause of disability—are common among people with disabilities and are the principal targets of health promotion and disease prevention efforts for this special population. Some, such as decubitus ulcers (pressure sores) and genitourinary disorders, are associated with living conditions linked to the disability, i.e., confinement to a wheel chair or bed. Immobility or inactivity also increases the risk of metabolic, circulatory, respiratory, and musculoskeletal problems.[7] Other secondary health problems can be seen as a progression of the original disabling condition. Diabetes, for example, can lead to serious foot problems and vision impairment.

Many secondary health problems are preventable. For others, the risks can be reduced. For example, pressure sores are a major health risk for all people with spinal cord injuries yet can be prevented through improved health care, properly designed seating, and personal hygiene. Remediable genitourinary tract disorders are also a problem for people whose major motor function is severely restricted. Inadequate health care is implicated in the development of these disorders. Other factors include nutritional disorders, alcohol and drug abuse, inadequate personal hygiene, and acute and chronic illness. Cardiovascular disorders and stroke, brought on by hypertension, nutritional problems, smoking, and lack of physical activity, may be particular problems for people with disabilities.[7]

Musculoskeletal disorders caused by a lack of physical activity and injuries are especially prevalent among people with disabilities. Many respiratory problems for people with disabilities are thought to be preventable. They can result from tobacco use, lack of physical activity, and inadequate immunization.

Alcohol and other drug abuse often are associated with emotional problems. For some people with disabilities, special risks may stem from negative family and cultural attitudes.

As with minority populations, the elements of this report that explicitly call for improvements for people with disabilities are limited by the availability of data with which to set targets. Disabilities vary in their type and their intensity; those with disabilities include all age, racial, and ethnic groups. One of the major challenges of the coming years is to improve our understanding of the needs of the full range of people with disabilities by improving the effectiveness of data systems.

Estimates of the number of people with chronic, significant disabilities vary from 34 million to 43 million. These estimates include the almost 4 percent of the total population of the Nation who are unable to perform their major activity (play, school, work, self-care); about 6 percent whose ability to perform major activities is limited in some fashion; and over 4 percent who are limited in nonmajor activities.[9] Many more people, of course, have impairments that are not yet, but could become, disabling; and still more have chronic conditions, such as hypertension or alcoholism, that can lead to impairment and disability. Many people have several disabling conditions. About 27 percent of people with disabilities report more than one cause of their limited function and over 7 percent report three or more.[9]

Activity limitations are most common among older people, the poor, and those Americans who are less educated. In comparison to the total population, about twice as many people in families with incomes of less than $10,000 a year report major activity limitation. Education too is clearly linked to disability; about 40 percent of people with 8 years or less of education have activity limitations compared to under 11 percent of those with 16 years or more.[9]

The prevalence of disability increases with age, as one would expect (Fig. 3.8). More than one out of every five people aged 65 and older is limited in one or more of his or her major activities, and nearly half of those aged 85 and older need assistance in activities of daily living. On the other hand, people who are under age 65 and living in the community, i.e., not institutionalized, make up about 40 percent of those who need assistance in activities of daily living.[9]

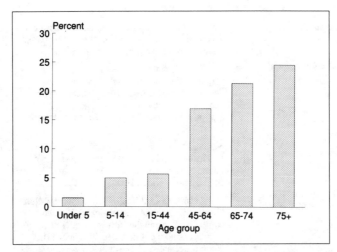

Fig. 3.8

Percentage of people experiencing limitation of major activity, by age (1987)

Source: *Health, United States, 1989 and Prevention Profile*

The major causes of activity limitation vary with age. People under age 18 are most likely to have disabilities associated with mental impairment, asthma, mental illness, deafness and other ear disorders, and speech impairments. Among young adults, orthopedic impairments, such as spinal curvature and other back impairments, are most common, while at older ages degenerative diseases, led by arthritis and heart disease, predominate.[9]

Among ethnic groups, American Indians have the highest rates of activity limitation and Asian and Pacific Islander Americans the lowest.[17] Activity limitations are slightly higher among blacks than among non-Hispanic whites, and both have higher rates of disability than Hispanics.

It is evident from this list that people with disabilities face many of the same risks as other people—nutritional problems, physical inactivity, alcohol and other drug abuse, and stress. But for people with disabilities reducing risks may be a particular challenge. Physical activity, considered especially important in preventing secondary health problems, offers a compelling example. To establish fitness regimens, people with disabilities often need to learn new skills, have access to special equipment, and be part of a support network that enables participation.[7]

Lack of adequate rehabilitation, maintenance therapies, and personal assistance increases the risk of secondary health problems among people with disabilities. Inadequate health insurance, especially among those without access to work-related group insurance, also poses a significant problem for this group.

A clear opportunity exists for health promotion and disease prevention efforts to improve the health prospects and functional independence of people with disabilities. Efforts to adapt existing preventive services and programs are underway. For example, exercise videotapes have been developed for people with paraplegia, quadriplegia, amputation, cerebral palsy, and other physical impairments. Some fitness centers offer modified aerobics, mild exercise in warm water, and other exercises designed to meet the needs of individuals with disabilities. But fitness services are just one of many that are needed. Preventing the occurrence of secondary health problems depends on the availability of a variety of health and social services. Gaps, overlaps, inconsistencies, and inequities in existing programs require the effective coordination of existing services if the health of people with disabilities is to be promoted.[7]

References

[1] Amler, R.W. and Dull, H.B., *Closing the Gap: The Burden of Unnecessary Illness.* New York: Oxford University Press, 1987.

[2] Asian American Health Forum. Year 2000 Strategic Health Development Program for Asian and Pacific Islander Americans. April 1989.

[3] Bureau of the Census. *U.S. Census of Population: 1980.* Washington DC: U.S. Department of Commerce.

[4] Council on Ethical and Judicial Affairs. Black-white disparities in health care. *JAMA* 263:2344-2346, 1990.

[5] Franks, A.L.; Berg, C.J.; Kane. M.A.; Browne, B.B.; et al. Hepatitis B virus infection among children born in the United States to Southeast Asian refugees, *New England Journal of Medicine* 321(9):1301-5, 1989.

[6] Indian Health Service, *Indian Health Service Chart Series Book,* Washington, DC: U.S. Department of Health and Human Services, 1988.

[7] Institute of Medicine. *Disability in America: A National Agenda.* edited by Pope, A. and Tarloff, A. Washington, DC: National Academy Press, in press.

[8] Institute of Medicine. *Preventing Low Birthweight.* Washington, DC: National Academy Press, 1985.

[9] LaPlante, M.P., *Data on Disability from the National Health Interview Survey, 1983-1985,* Washington, D.C.: National Institute on Disability and Rehabilitation Research, 1988.

[10] National Cancer Institute and National Center for Health Statistics. Unpublished data from the Cancer Control Supplement to the 1987 National Health Interview Survey.

[11] National Center for Children in Poverty. *A Statistical Profile of Our Poorest Young Citizens.* New York: the Center, 1990.

[12] National Center for Health Statistics. *Health, United States, 1989 and Prevention Profile.* Hyattsville, MD: U.S. Department of Health and Human Services, 1990.

[13] National Coalition of Hispanic Health and Human Services Organizations. *Delivering Preventive Health Care to Hispanics: A Manual for Providers,* Washington, DC: the Coaltion, 1988.

[14] National Health and Nutrition Examination Survey (NHANES) II, National Center for Health Statistics, Centers for Disease Control, Public Health Service, U.S. Department of Health and Human Services, Hyattsville, MD.

[15] National Health Interview Survey, National Center for Health Statistics, Centers for Disease Control, Public Health Service, U.S. Department of Health and Human Service, Hyattsville, MD.

[16] National Heart, Lung, and Blood Institute, National Cholesterol Education Program. *Report of the Expert Panel on Population Strategies for Blood Cholesterol Reduction.* Washington, DC: U.S. Department of Health and Human Services, 1990.

[17] National Institute on Disability and Rehabilitation Research, *Chartbook on Disability in the United States,* Washington, DC: the Institute 1989.

[18] National Migrant Resource Program and the Migrant Clinicians Network. *Migrant and Seasonal Farmworker, Health Objectives for the Year 2000: Document in Progress, April 1990.* Austin, TX: National Migrant Resource Program, Inc., 1990.

[19] National Vital Statistics System, National Center for Health Statistics, Centers for Disease Control, Public Health Service, U.S. Department of Health and Human Services, Hyattsville, MD.

[20] North Carolina Oral Health School Survey. North Carolina Division of Dental Health, Raleigh, North Carolina and the University of North Carolina School of Public Health, Chapel Hill, North Carolina.

[21] Office on Smoking and Health. Unpublished data from the 1987 National Health Interview Survey.

[22] Office of Substance Abuse Prevention (OSAP). Communicating about alcohol and other drugs: Strategies for reaching populations at risk. *OSAP Prevention Monograph 4.* Washington, DC: U.S. Department of Health and Human Services, in press.

[23] Public Health Service. *The Surgeon General's Report on Nutrition and Health.* Washington, DC: U.S. Department of Health and Human Services, 1988.

[24] Rhoades, E.R.; Hammond, J.; Welty, T.K.; Handler, A.O.; and Amler, R.W. The Indian burden of illness and future health interventions. *Public Health Reports 102(4):*361-8, 1987.

[25] Schwartz, S.M. and Thomas, D.B. "Estimates of Cancer Incidence Among Southeast Asian Refugees in the United States." Paper presented at the Annual Meeting of the American Public Health Association, New Orleans, LA October 1987.

[26] Selik, R.M.; Castro, K.G.; and Papaionnou, M. Racial/ethnic differences in the risk of AIDS in the United States. *American Journal of Public Health* 78(12):1539-1544, 1988.

[27] Selik, R.M.; Castro, K.G.; Papaionnou, M.; and Ruehler, J.W. Birthplace and the risk of AIDS among Hispanics in the United States. *American Journal of Public Health* 79(7):836-9, 1989.

[28] Smith, J.C.; Mercy, J.A.; and Rosenberg, M.L. Suicide and homicide among Hispanics in the Southwest. *Public Health Reports* 101(3):265-270, 1986.

[29] Subcommittee on Definition and Prevalence, Joint National Committee on Detection, Evaluation, and Treatment of High Blood Pressure. Hypertension prevalance and the status of awareness, treatment and control. *Hypertension* 7(3):460, 1985.

[30] U.S. Department of Health and Human Services. *Report of the Secretary's Task Force on Black and Minority Health.* Washington, DC: the Department, 1985.

4. Goals for the Nation

The promise embodied in *Healthy People 2000* involves people in all their variety: age, gender, family relationships, racial and ethnic identity, income level, education, and occupation. It involves birth and death, two sentinel health events. Birth frames the potential for a healthy lifetime; death often summarizes how that potential was used. It involves the values of family, neighborhood, community, and Nation, enabling or undermining the health course that a life takes. It involves an array of risks—some posing apparent, immediate danger and others invisible and delayed in their effects. Finally, it involves medical science and medical care, with their ability to thwart infections, reverse the course of some chronic diseases, and enhance ability to function where limitations exist.

Three overarching goals emerge from the complexity of the health challenge of the 1990s. They permeate the structure and the content of this report. They further define the challenge, especially for health planners, policy-makers, and providers (Fig. 4.1).

* **Increase the span of healthy life for Americans**
* **Reduce health disparities among Americans**
* **Achieve access to preventive services for all Americans**

Fig. 4.1

Healthy People 2000 Goals

Goal I
Increase the Span of Healthy Life for Americans

A central purpose of *Healthy People 2000* is to increase the proportion of Americans who live long and healthy lives. The first goal underlying our strategy for the coming decade clearly states this intention. It encompasses the essential elements of health promotion and disease prevention: prevention of premature death, disability, and disease, and enhancement of the quality of life.

From an individual perspective, healthy life extends into the final quarter of a full century, free from chronic, disabling diseases and conditions, from preventable infections, and from serious injury. It means a full range of functional capacity at each life stage, from infancy through old age, allowing one the ability to enter into satisfying relationships with others, to work, and to play. From a national perspective, healthy life means a vital, creative, and productive citizenry contributing to thriving communities and a thriving Nation.

In the course of this century, average life expectancy at birth has increased by almost 60 percent, from 47 years in 1900 to 75 years in 1987 (Fig. 4.2). This progress has been largely due to the advances of science and public health in conquering life-threatening communicable diseases. The aging of the population and the evolution from communicable diseases to chronic diseases and injuries as the leading causes of death and disability direct our attention to quality of life issues. Both chronic diseases and injuries can be measured by the death certificates that they generate; but the numbers reflecting human suffering and costs associated with heart disease, cancer, nonfatal strokes, diabetes, and lung diseases far outstrip mortality statistics. The results of injury caused both by unintentional trauma and by interpersonal violence are not limited to lives cut short; they also include lives that must overcome brain damage, motor limitations, and other permanent impairments.

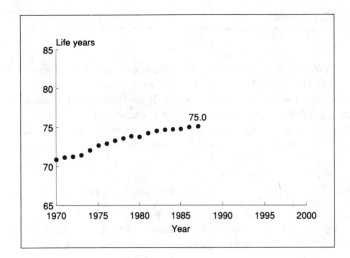

Fig. 4.2

Life expectancy at birth, U.S. population

Source: *Health, United States, 1989 and Prevention Profile*

We can measure our progress in increasing the span of healthy life in several ways. One measure offered here indicates the rate of deaths per 100,000 people before age 75, the approximate average life expectancy at birth in 1990 (Fig. 4.3). Infant mortality, a traditional tool for judging the effectiveness and compassion of health systems, can indicate national progress at the early end of the age spectrum (Fig. 4.4).

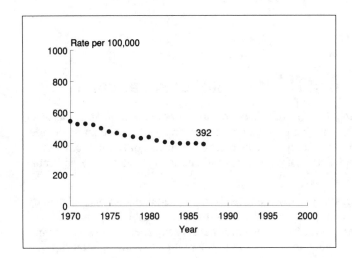

Fig. 4.3

Death rates for people aged 74 and younger, U.S. population (age-adjusted)

Source: National Vital Statistics System (CDC)

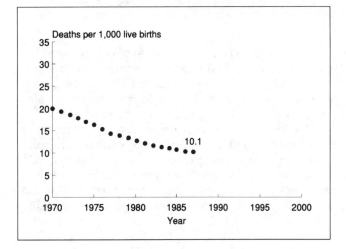

Fig. 4.4

Infant mortality rate, U.S. population

Source: National Vital Statistics System (CDC)

Another measure uses a formula that combines death rates with acute and chronic illnesses, impairments, and handicaps to define average years of healthy life. Using this measure, time spent in a healthy state or years of healthy life can be compared to the average life expectancy at birth. (Fig. 4.5) The difference between these two estimates indicates the average amount of time spent in a dysfunctional state due to either chronic or acute limitation. One major indicator of dysfunction is limitation of major activity due to chronic conditions. (Fig. 4.6) Years of healthy life uses a life expectancy model in which standard life table data are adjusted for level of well-being of a population. Measures of well-being represent individual functioning and include measures of mental, physical, and social functioning. For example, social functioning may be measured in terms of an individual's limitation in performing his or her usual social role, whether this be work, school, or housework; physical functioning may be measured in terms of being confined to bed, chair, or couch due to health reasons, or in terms of health-related limitation in mobility. Because years of healthy life is a relatively new type of measure, the baseline estimates may change. Nonetheless it should prove an informative indicator as we track the Nation's health progress.

Over the course of the decade, we will be able to use each of these measures as indicators of our overall progress in increasing the span of healthy life. To explain the basis for that progress, it is necessary to move beyond the broad goals that are proposed here and look to the priorities for preventive action. Healthy life will be expanded to more years and more Americans as a result of efforts to address the priorities defined in the next chapter.

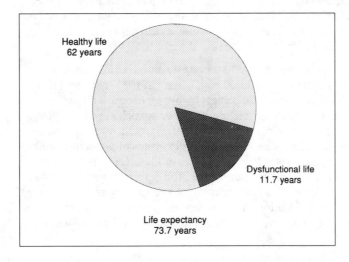

Fig. 4.5

Years of healthy life as a proportion of life expectancy, U.S. population (1980)

Source: National Vital Statistics System and National Health Interview Survey (CDC)

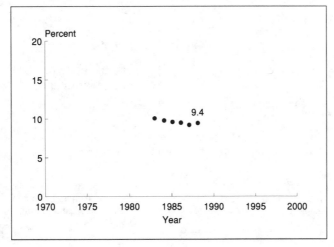

Fig. 4.6

Percentage of people experiencing limitation of major activity, U.S. population (crude rates)

Source: National Health Interview Survey (CDC)

Goal II
Reduce Health Disparities Among Americans

Achieving a healthier America depends on significant improvements in the health of population groups that now are at highest risk of premature death, disease, and disability. The particular health problems of those high risk groups were presented in the previous two chapters. In some instances and for some health risks, they are age groups. In most cases and for virtually all health risks, they are members of certain racial and ethnic groups, people with low income, and people with disabilities. Special attention is needed to close the gap that exists between the majority of the population and the various minority populations. Whether the issue is chronic diseases, infectious diseases, unintentional injuries, or violence-related injuries, the services and protection that might most effectively bring about improvements in their circumstances must be made available.

Although health statistics that take race and ethnicity into account are sparse, the ones that do exist leave no doubt about disparities. The greatest opportunities for improvement and the greatest threats to the future health status of the Nation reside in population groups that have historically been disadvantaged economically, educationally, and politically. These must be our first priority.

Even as average life expectancy at birth edged into the upper 70s, the expected life span for black American male babies born in 1986, 1987, and 1988 actually shrank.[1] The disparities appear across the spectrum of health concerns, not just in average life expectancy. (Fig. 4.7) One perspective on these differences is death rates before age 75 (Fig. 4.8). A particularly sensitive and compelling measure of disparity is infant mortality. Although America's infant mortality rate is at an all-time low, a persistent racial gap remains. Black babies continue to die at twice the rate of white babies (Fig. 4.9).

Another is potential years of life lost before age 65 among white and black men from chronic diseases, calculated as years lost per 1,000 population. In 1987, rates for black men are 55 percent higher for heart disease, 26 percent higher for cancer, 180 percent higher for stroke, and 100 percent higher for lung disease. For homicide, years of potential life lost were 630 percent higher for black men than for white men. Among women of both races, death rates for all causes were lower, but comparisons of premature death of white and black women are equally startling. Lost years of life before age 65 were 134 percent higher among black women for heart disease, 166 percent higher for stroke, and 360 percent higher for homicide.[1] Statistics to compute years of potential life lost are scarce for other racial and ethnic populations, for low-income groups, and for people with disabilities, but analyses of local data from small area studies confirm disparities among these groups as well.

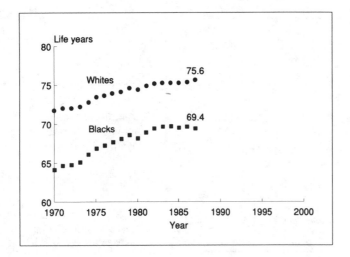

Fig. 4.7

Life expectancy at birth, blacks and whites

Source: *Health, United States, 1989 and Prevention Profile*

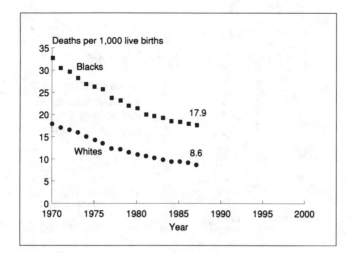

Fig. 4.8

Infant mortality rates, blacks and whites

Source: National Vital Statistics System and National Linked Birth and Infant Death Data Set (CDC)

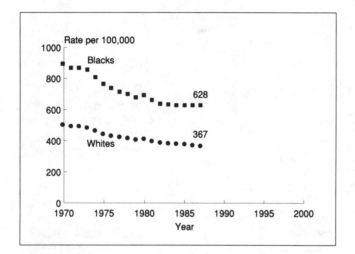

Fig. 4.9

Death rates for people aged 74 and younger, blacks and whites (1987)

Source: National Vital Statistics System (CDC)

Contrasting death rates are mirrored by statistics that depict disability outcome, as well as death. Statistics on years of healthy life reflect the gap between our racial and ethnic groups in the United States (Fig. 4.10). Similarly, rates of disability, measured in terms of limitation of major activity, confirm the fact of inequity in health. The most striking aspect of these comparative rates is the great gap between low-income people and all other groups (Fig. 4.11).

Healthy People 2000 thus calls for special attention to reducing—and finally eliminating—disparities among population groups of Americans. In the priorities for preventive action, this report sets separate, challenging targets when baseline data are available. Usually the targets are sufficient to narrow the gap between the death, disease, or disability rates for population groups and the total population; where trends have been worsening for population groups, targets may appear less challenging but may, in fact, be difficult to achieve because of recent setbacks. In many instances, targets cannot be set in 1990 because measurement tools are not available to provide baselines from which to set realistic, achievable targets for 2000. For this reason, the health status of black Americans, for whom data are most readily available, is used to provide proxy measures of our progress in moving toward the basic goal of equity in health for all our Nation's people.

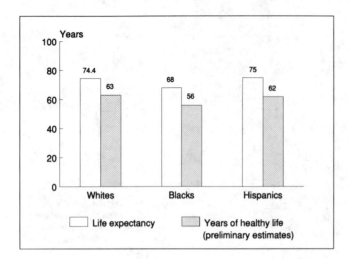

Fig. 4.10

Life expectancy and years of healthy life, whites, blacks, and Hispanics (1980)

Source: Analysis based on data from the National Vital Statistics System (CDC), National Health Interview Survey (CDC), and the U.S. Census Bureau

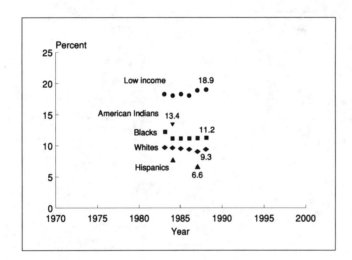

Fig. 4.11

Percentage of people experiencing limitation of major activity, by race and ethnicity (crude rates)

Source: National Health Interview Survey (CDC)

Goal III
Achieve Access to Preventive Services for All Americans

Healthy People 2000 calls for a comprehensive strategy to support the improvements in health that are possible through prevention. This report defines the major parts of that strategy as Health Promotion, Health Protection, and Preventive Services. The priorities for prevention are grouped under these three categories. They are not precise or mutually exclusive categories, but they serve to underscore an important point. Major improvements depend on all three approaches to prevention, not just one. We cannot rely solely on success in persuading people to change their health-related behaviors through health promotion efforts, any more than we can rely solely on environmental improvements or expanded and enhanced clinical interventions.

A health strategy for the 1990s, however, must put particular emphasis on the arena where health professionals in both the private and public sectors have most responsibility, namely the arena of preventive services. Those services, made available to all Americans, can provide the foundation for achievement of other parts of our health strategy. An example, which we will use to track our effectiveness in moving toward this goal, relates to the birth of healthy babies. Prenatal health care is a vital, fundamental ingredient in attaining this sentinel health event (Fig. 4.12). Early and regular prenatal visits to qualified health care providers can ensure greater likelihood that low birth weight and other perinatal complications will be prevented. Prenatal health care services can also serve as a resource and a reinforcer for health promotion efforts that are equally important to healthy pregnancies. The role of prenatal services in education and counseling about parental behaviors, including nutrition, abstinence from tobacco, alcohol, and other drugs, and, even before conception, behaviors that involve risks of sexually transmitted diseases, including HIV infection, is crucial. Likewise, preventive services for pregnant women can serve as the means of monitoring protection against toxic exposures, such as lead, dangerous prescription medications, and radiation.

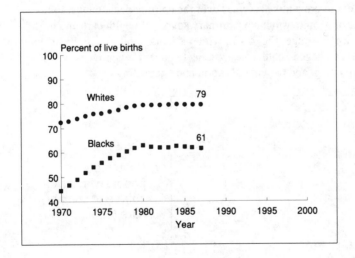

Fig. 4.12

Percentage of pregnant women receiving first trimester prenatal care, blacks and whites

Source: National Vital Statistics System (CDC)

Other preventive services are equally fundamental to our national prevention plan. Basic monitoring of child growth and development; immunization against childhood diseases (Fig. 4.13); appropriate immunization for vulnerable adults against pneumonia and influenza; screening to detect high blood pressure and high blood cholesterol and breast, cervical, oropharyngeal, and colorectal cancers; counseling on nutrition, smoking cessation, and injury prevention; all these services are indispensable parts of prevention. Achievement of this goal clearly requires that health care providers offer, and patients receive, these services. Objectives throughout this report focus on increasing the proportion of primary care providers who routinely offer preventive services to their patients.

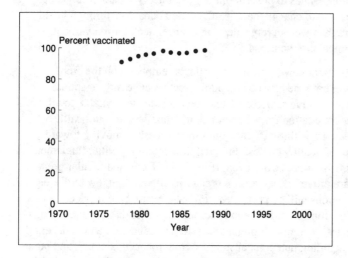

Fig. 4.13

Percentage of children immunized by time of school entry

Source: Center for Prevention Services, CDC

Access to preventive services involves more than just availability of services. Preventive services cannot, and should not, be separated from basic primary health care. Approximately 18 percent of all Americans and 31 percent of those without either private or public health insurance have no source of primary health care. (Fig. 4.14) Thus, tracking of progress to achieve access to preventive services over the coming decade must focus on increases in the number of people who have a primary source of health care and those who have adequate insurance coverage (Fig. 4.15), with particular attention to the extension of health insurance and managed health care systems to cover preventive services such as immunizations, screening, and patient education and counseling.

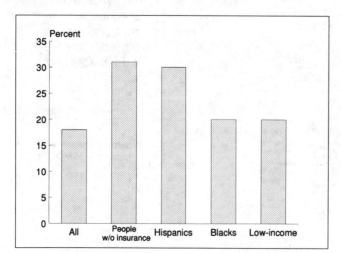

Fig. 4.14

Percentage of people who lack a source of primary care (1986)

Source: Robert Wood Johnson Foundation

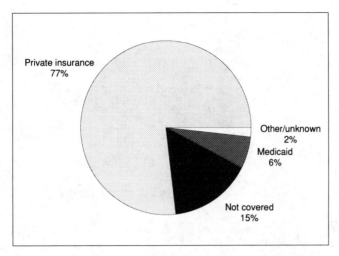

Fig. 4.15

Health insurance coverage for people aged 64 and younger, by type of coverage (1986)

Source: Based on *Health, United States, 1989 and Prevention Profile*

Note: Percent distribution approximate due to overlap among categories.

These three goals—healthy lives for more Americans, elimination of disparities among population groups, access to necessary preventive services for everyone—are our broad national aspirations for health improvements. They can serve as a shared set of values that underpin all of our health promotion and disease prevention work. They can inform our public policy, whether at the Federal, State, or local levels. But taken alone, they do not provide us with adequate direction to guide actual decisions about programs, resource allocation, or professional and personal commitments. The goals are insufficient, unless they are buttressed by a framework of specific and substantive preventive actions that will move us steadily in the direction of their achievement. The next chapter lays out the specifics of the *Healthy People 2000* plan and gives substance to the goals for the Nation.

Reference

[1] National Center for Health Statistics. *Health, United States, 1989 and Prevention Profile*. DHHS Pub. No. (PHS)90-1232. Hyattsville, MD: U.S. Department of Health and Human Services, 1990.

5. Priorities for Health Promotion and Disease Prevention

Healthy People 2000 is a platform for action. The information it contains may be interesting; the statistical data on which it is based may be analytically useful; and the objectives-oriented structure that it employs may serve as a practical model for other planning endeavors. But its value must finally be judged by how well it helps to shape what we do to improve the health of the Nation in the coming decade.

This chapter summarizes the priorities for preventive action. Organized in three basic categories—Health Promotion, Health Protection, and Preventive Services—it outlines specific behavioral risks, disease conditions, and health outcomes that must be effectively addressed in the coming years if we are to take advantage of our opportunities for better health. In addition, a cross-cutting priority that supports each of the others is improvement of our surveillance and data systems to foster more effective decision-making.

Each specific priority is summarized in the following pages, together with representative health objectives drawn from Part II of *Healthy People 2000*. These representative objectives serve as abbreviated examples of the measurable targets that are more fully stated and discussed in greater detail in Part II. While they cannot completely summarize all aspects of the health improvements, risk reductions, and service enhancements that are contained in the chapters of Part II, these examples demonstrate the magnitude and importance of the change envisioned in *Healthy People 2000*.

Health Promotion

Physical Activity and Fitness

Nutrition

Tobacco

Alcohol and Other Drugs

Family Planning

Mental Health and Mental Disorders

Violent and Abusive Behavior

Educational and Community-Based Programs

Physical Activity and Fitness

Regular physical activity increases life expectancy,[74] can help older adults maintain functional independence, and enhances quality of life at each stage of life.[33] The beneficial impact of physical activity touches widely on various diseases and conditions. Regular physical activity can help to prevent and manage coronary heart disease, hypertension, diabetes, osteoporosis, and depression.[26] It has also been associated with a lower rate of colon cancer[77] and stroke[83], and may be linked to reduced back injury.[8] It is an essential component of weight loss programs.

Physical activity is a complex behavior and its relationship with health is multifaceted. Regular vigorous physical activity promotes cardiorespiratory fitness and helps prevent coronary heart disease.[5,75] Activity that builds muscular strength, endurance, and flexibility may protect against injury and disability. And any activity that expends energy is important in weight control. Physical activity can also produce changes in blood pressure, blood lipids, clotting factors, and glucose tolerance, that may help prevent and control high blood pressure, coronary heart disease and diabetes.[38]

While activity should be habitual, it need not be unduly strenuous. People who engage daily in light to moderate exercise, equivalent to sustained walking for about 30 minutes a day, can achieve substantial health gains. Increasing evidence suggests that even small increases in light to moderate activity by those who are least active will produce measurable health benefits.[39,82]

Of particular importance is the role of physical activity in preventing coronary heart disease, the leading cause of death in the United States. A sedentary lifestyle appears to be an independent risk factor for coronary heart disease, nearly doubling a person's risk.[78] Its effect on coronary heart disease risk is almost as great as the better known risk factors, such as cigarette smoking and high blood pressure. Because more people are at risk of coronary heart disease due to physical inactivity than to any other single risk factor, it has an especially great public health impact.

Few Americans engage in regular physical activity despite the potential benefits. Currently, only 22 percent of adults engage in at least 30 minutes of light to moderate physical activity 5 or more times per week, and only 12 percent report that they are this active 7 or more times a week. Less than 10 percent of the population exercises 3 or more times a week at the more vigorous level necessary to improve cardiorespiratory fitness. Nearly 25 percent of adults report no leisure-time physical activity, and the prevalence of sedentary behavior increases with advancing age.

To increase physical activity and fitness, by the year 2000...

**1.3   Increase moderate daily physical activity to at least 30% of people
(a 36% increase)**

**1.5   Reduce sedentary lifestyles to no more than 15% of people
(a 38% decrease)**

Other objectives target sustained combined changes in diet and activity patterns for those who are overweight; physical education in schools; sponsorship by employers of worksite physical activity programs; increasing accessibility of community resources like trails and pools; and a stronger focus by primary care providers on the physical activity patterns of their patients.

Nutrition

In ways often interrelated with patterns of physical inactivity, dietary factors are associated with 5 of the 10 leading causes of death in the United States: coronary heart disease, some types of cancer, stroke, noninsulin-dependent diabetes mellitus, and atherosclerosis. The 1988 *Surgeon General's Report on Nutrition and Health*[79] found that for the 2 out of 3 Americans who neither smoke nor drink, eating patterns may shape their long-term health prospects more than any other personal choice. In general, excesses and imbalances of some food components in the diet have replaced once-prevalent nutrient deficiencies as the principal concern.

While many dietary components are involved in diet and health relationships, chief among them is the disproportionate consumption of foods high in fats (especially saturated fats), often at the expense of foods high in complex carbohydrates and dietary fiber that may be more conducive to health.[79] To help promote health and prevent chronic disease, the *Dietary Guidelines for Americans*,[91] issued by the United States Departments of Health and Human Services and Agriculture, recommend one should eat a variety of foods; maintain healthy weight; choose a diet low in fat, saturated fat, and cholesterol; choose a diet with plenty of vegetables, fruits, and grain products; use sugars only in moderation; use salt and sodium only in moderation; and, if alcoholic beverages are consumed, do so in moderation.

Overweight affects about 26 percent of the population. It is a particular problem for poor and minority populations, affecting 44 percent of black women over age 20 and 37 percent of all women below the poverty level. Obesity has been linked to increased risk for diabetes mellitus, high blood pressure and stroke, coronary heart disease, some types of cancer, and gallbladder disease.[79]

Dietary fat contributes more than twice as many calories per unit of weight as carbohydrate or protein, and currently constitutes 36 percent of the calories in the average American diet. Considerable evidence associates diets high in fat with increased risk of obesity, some types of cancer, and possibly gallbladder disease.[79] Strong and consistent evidence relates saturated fat intake to high blood cholesterol and increased risk for coronary heart disease. Moreover, Americans eat only about half of the dietary fiber recommended by the National Cancer Institute to help reduce the risk for some types of cancer. Dietary fiber is readily available from a variety of foods such as vegetables, fruits, and grains, which are also low in fat.

To improve nutrition, by the year 2000...

2.3   Reduce overweight to a prevalence of no more than 20% of people (a 23% decrease)

2.5   Reduce dietary fat intake to an average of 30% of calories (a 17% decrease)

Other objectives target increasing consumption of vegetables, fruits, and grain products; decreasing sodium consumption; increasing calcium intake, in particular for young people and pregnant or lactating women; increasing breastfeeding; reducing iron deficiency and growth retardation in children; useful and informative nutrition labeling for all food products; increasing availability of low-fat products; better identification of low-fat, low-calorie food choices in restaurants; more attention to nutrition education and food choices in schools; better use of worksites for nutrition education and services; and a stronger focus by primary care providers on the nutritional practices of their patients.

Tobacco

Tobacco use is the most important single preventable cause of death in the United States, accounting for one of every six deaths, or some 390,000 deaths annually.[73] It is a major risk factor for diseases of the heart and blood vessels; chronic bronchitis and emphysema; cancers of the lung, larynx, pharynx, oral cavity, esophagus, pancreas, and bladder; and other problems such as respiratory infections and stomach ulcers.[73] Cigarette smoking is responsible for an estimated 21 percent of all coronary heart disease deaths (40 percent of those under age 65), 30 percent of all cancer deaths, and 87 percent of lung cancer deaths in the United States. The risk of dying from lung cancer is 22 times higher for men and 12 times higher for women who smoke than for lifetime nonsmokers. Passive or involuntary smoking causes lung cancer and other diseases in healthy nonsmokers and severe respiratory problems in children. Middle ear infections in children have been linked to passive smoking.

Cigarette smoking during pregnancy is a risk factor for low birth weight, prematurity, miscarriage, sudden infant death syndrome, and other maternal and infant health problems. Between 20 and 30 percent of the incidence of low birth weight,[36] up to 14 percent of preterm deliveries, and about 10 percent of all infant deaths are attributable to maternal cigarette smoking.[73] Yet 25 percent of pregnant women smoke throughout their pregnancy.[50]

Cigarette smoking has declined dramatically since 1964, when the first Surgeon General's report on smoking appeared. In 1987, 29 percent of adults smoked compared to 40 percent in 1965. Nearly half of all living adults who ever smoked have quit. Nevertheless, smoking rates remain high in certain populations, including blacks, blue collar workers, and people with fewer years of education. In 1987, 34 percent of blacks smoked.[73] Smoking is a special problem for workers with exposure to hazardous substances that may compound the risk.

Among youth, more than half of 8th graders and nearly two-thirds of 10th graders report having tried cigarettes.[4] More than one-fourth of 10th graders report having smoked a cigarette during the preceding month and nearly one in five reports smoking a pack or more in the previous month.

To reduce use of tobacco, by the year 2000...

3.4 **Reduce cigarette smoking prevalence to no more than 15% of adults (a 48% decrease)**

3.5 **Reduce initiation of smoking to no more than 15% by age 20 (a 50% decrease)**

Other objectives target reducing lung cancer and chronic obstructive lung disease deaths; increasing smoking cessation during pregnancy; reducing use of smokeless tobacco; prevention education and tobacco-free environments in schools; restrictions on smoking in the workplace and other public places; enforcement of prohibition of sales of tobacco products to youth; restrictions on tobacco advertising and promotion targeting youth; State plans to reduce tobacco use; and more smoking cessation assistance to patients by primary care providers.

Alcohol and Other Drugs

Approximately two-thirds of American adults drink alcohol at least occasionally. Of these, it is estimated that about 18 million currently experience problems as a result of alcohol use, and about 7 percent of drinkers experience moderate levels of dependence symptoms.[65] Alcohol is a factor in approximately half of all homicides, suicides, and motor vehicle fatalities.[76] With fetal alcohol syndrome affecting as many as 3 infants per 1,000 live births in some hospital reports, it is the leading preventable cause of birth defects.[65] Alcohol is also responsible for numerous deaths due to liver disease. Of special concern are the problems for young people. Nine out of ten high school seniors report using alcohol at least once.

Drug use is also a dominant societal concern. Surveys in 1988 found that 21 million Americans had used cocaine at least once, and 21 million also had used marijuana in the last year.[63] Among high school seniors, almost 44 percent report having tried marijuana, and 10 percent report ever using cocaine.[45] It has been estimated that one in four American adolescents is at very high risk of alcohol and other drug problems and their consequences.[20] The data may underestimate the problem because existing surveys fail to count high risk youth who have dropped out of school. Drug abuse is linked to high rates of violent crime in the Nation, to transmission of the HIV virus, and to developmental problems in infants.

These are the immediate health problems posed by alcohol and other drugs. Their abuse, however, is closely related to a host of other social and health problems, such as early unwanted pregnancy, delinquency, and school failure. The economic cost of problems attendant to alcohol abuse was estimated in 1990 to be $70 billion, and another $44 billion for drug problems.[27,80] Alcohol and other drug abuse appears to be declining across the total population. Use of crack cocaine, however, is on the rise, especially in some urban centers. Homeless people are at special risk of alcohol abuse.[64]

In the past decade, public awareness of this problem grew, uniting diverse groups in the common goal. Businesses, schools, parent groups, and minority organizations have developed ways to fight the pervasive dangers of alcohol and other drugs. A changing social climate has been accompanied by legislative and policy actions, particularly concerning drinking and driving.

To reduce alcohol and other drug abuse, by the year 2000...

4.1 **Reduce alcohol-related motor vehicle crash deaths to no more than 8.5 per 100,000 people (age adjusted)**
(a 12% decrease)

4.6 **Reduce alcohol use by school children aged 12 to 17 to less than 13%; marijuana use by youth aged 18 to 25 to less than 8%; and cocaine use by youth aged 18 to 25 to less than 3%**
(50% decreases)

Other objectives target increasing the average age of first use of addictive substances; reducing occasions of heavy drinking by young people; reducing aggregate per capita alcohol consumption nationally; increasing awareness of the harmful effects of addictive substances; better access to treatment programs; stronger and better enforced laws related to driving under the influence of intoxicants; better access of workers to assistance for problems; policies to reduce minors' access to alcohol; and greater involvement of primary care providers in dealing with these problems.

Family Planning

Families are the bedrock of our society. Decisions about forming a family are of critical importance. Decisions made today may have long-term consequences. Safe and healthful childbearing both contributes to, and is a result of, effective family planning. Miscarriage, stillbirth, and infant mortality are tragic examples of problems that occur more frequently as a result of family planning failures. Family planning is defined here as the process of establishing the preferred number and spacing of children in one's family and selecting the means by which these preferences are achieved. It presupposes the importance of family and the importance of planning. It requires that fundamental questions be addressed concerning an individual's relationship to the lives, health, and well-being of others.

Successful implementation of family planning choices requires mature, thoughtful decisions accompanied by motivation to carry out those decisions. It requires the exercise of personal responsibility. There are many effective means by which family planning choices can be implemented. Childbearing, adoption, abstinence from sexual activity outside of a monogamous relationship, use of contraception methods, natural family planning, and treatment of infertility are all means of reaching desired family planning goals.

Despite the fundamental importance of these decisions to each individual and to society as a whole, problems attendant to poor family planning exert a tremendous toll on our Nation. In 1988, nearly half of American women surveyed reported that their pregnancies in the last 5 years had been mistimed or unwanted—56 percent if adjustment is made for unreported abortions.[69]

The problem is most pressing among young people. More than three out of four young women and 85 percent of young men have had sexual intercourse by age 20.[69,87] Each year, one out of ten young women in this age group becomes pregnant. By age 20, approximately 40 percent of all women have been pregnant while 63 percent of black women have been pregnant.[90] An estimated 84 percent of these pregnancies were unintended,[32] and abortion rates among American teenagers are considerably higher than for many other countries.

To improve family planning, by the year 2000...

5.1 Reduce teenage pregnancies to no more than 50 per 1,000 girls aged 17 and younger (a 30% decrease)

5.2 Reduce unintended pregnances to no more than 30% of pregnancies (a 46% decrease)

Other objectives target reducing sexual intercourse among teenagers; reducing nonuse of contraceptives among those who are unmarried and sexually active; increasing effectiveness with which contraceptives are used; improving communication between adolescents and parents on human sexuality; increasing availability of appropriate preconception counseling; increasing referral rates to appropriate services; increasing availability of information on adoption for unmarried pregnant patients; and reducing rates of infertility.

Mental Health and Mental Disorders

Mental health refers to an individual's ability to negotiate the daily challenges and social interactions of life, without experiencing undue emotional or behavioral incapacity. It can be affected by numerous factors ranging from exogenous stresses presenting in ways that may be difficult to manage to organic disease or genetic defects that impair brain function. An estimated 23 million noninstitutionalized adults in the United States have cognitive, emotional, or behavioral disorders, not including alcohol and other drug abuse. Schizophrenic disorders most often result in functional disabilities, but depression is the most common of the major disorders, affecting about 5 percent of the population at any one time.

Suicide is clearly the most serious of the potential outcomes of these disorders and it claims more than 30,000 lives each year.[70] Injuries from firearms are directly responsible for a majority of suicidal deaths, and much of the increase in suicide that has taken place since the 1950s is specific to firearm deaths.[6,46] There has been a steady increase in deaths from suicide among youth aged 15 to 19, and by the mid-1980s suicide was the second leading cause of death in this age group.

A variety of approaches have been proposed to reduce the impact of mental health problems. Stress, whether stemming from life events, chronic strain, or environmental pressures, is associated with biological changes linked to cognitive, emotional, and behavioral dysfunctions. Healthful habits, such as good nutrition and adequate amounts of exercise, and relaxation techniques may be useful in helping to relieve stress. Because people with low levels of control over their environment (actual or perceived) appear to be at greater risk, interventions have also been directed at increasing individuals' resources and coping skills through education and social support. For those needing more aggressive attention, medical interventions are available that include antidepression drugs, psychotherapeutic agents, and biofeedback.

Childhood developmental delays and specific skill disorders have also been linked to learning and adjustment problems in adolescence and early adulthood. Early interventions with parents and children that address prenatal care, parental skills, and remedial help in early school programs may help prevent developmental problems and their progression to mental health problems.

To improve mental health and prevent mental disorders, by the year 2000...

**6.1   Reduce suicides to no more than 10.5 per 100,000 people
(a 10% decrease)**

**6.5   Reduce adverse effects of stress to less than 35% of people
(an 18% decrease)**

Other objectives target reducing prevalence of mental disorders; increasing utilization of community support programs; increasing treatment for those with major depressive disorders; increasing use of broad social support mechanisms for those with trouble coping; more attention by employers to services related to managing employee stress; better access to mutual-help clearinghouses; and more attention by primary care providers to the cognitive, emotional, and behavioral needs of their patients.

Violent and Abusive Behavior

Violent and abusive behavior (intentional injury) exacts a large toll on the physical and mental health of Americans. Child abuse, spouse abuse, and other forms of intrafamilial violence continue to threaten the health of thousands of American families. Homicide and suicide account for over one-third of the more than 145,000 injury deaths that occur in the United States each year. Because of its growing prominence as a source of the leading health problems experienced by Americans, violent and abusive behavior has been increasingly recognized as an important public health problem.

Homicide is the 11th leading cause of death in the United States, accounting for nearly 21,000 deaths in 1987.[51] Men, teenagers, young adults, and minority group members, particularly blacks and Hispanics, are most likely to be murder victims. It is the leading cause of death for blacks between the ages of 15 and 34.[13] Overall homicide rates for blacks have declined since 1970, while the rates for whites have increased.[13] Most homicides are committed with a firearm, occur during an argument, and occur among people who are acquainted with one another. Homicide rates in the United States far exceed those of any other developed country.

Assault injuries are another consequence of interpersonal violence. Each year between 1979 and 1986 more than 2.2 million people suffered nonfatal injuries from violent and abusive behavior. Of these injured victims, 1 million received medical care and 500,000 were treated by emergency medical facilities.[25] More than 25 percent of the Nation's 10,000 to 15,000 spinal cord injuries each year are the result of assaultive violence. Firearms account for 60 percent of all homicides and suicides, and a substantial proportion of all traumatic spinal cord injuries.[44]

Intrafamilial violence is more prevalent than often recognized. In 1986 an estimated 1.6 million children nationwide experienced some form of abuse or neglect.[95] Physical abuse accounted for the greatest portion of abuse incidents, followed by emotional and then sexual abuse. Studies also suggest that between 2 and 4 million women are physically battered each year by partners including husbands, former husbands, boyfriends, and lovers. Between 21 and 30 percent of all women in the United States are estimated to have been beaten by a partner at least once. More than 1 million women seek medical assistance for injuries caused by battering each year, and the vast majority of domestic homicides are preceded by episodes of violence.[56]

To reduce violent and abusive behavior, by the year 2000...

**7.1   Reduce homicides to no more than 7.2 per 100,000 people
(a 15% decrease)**

**7.6   Reduce assault injuries to no more than 10 per 1,000 people
(a 10% decrease)**

Other objectives target reducing weapon-related injury deaths; reducing child and spouse abuse, reducing rape; reducing weapon-carrying by adolescents; reducing inappropriate storage of weapons; improving emergency treatment, housing, and referral services for battered women, children, and older people; improving school programs for conflict resolution; and strengthening State-based efforts in violence prevention.

Educational and Community-Based Programs

A supportive social environment may be the most important factor in changing behaviors that contribute to many of today's leading health threats. Consequently activity and leadership at the community level is fundamental to progress. Educational and community-based programs, developed to reach people outside of traditional health care settings, may address one risk factor in one setting, but increasingly they use multiple interventions in a variety of settings.

Many involve various sectors and levels of society. Changes in the social and physical environment call for the involvement of social institutions, businesses, legislative and judicial bodies, the media, and other parts of the community. Because comprehensive, communitywide programs aim to draw upon and become involved in as many aspects of community life as possible, they require a high degree of cooperation and coordination between groups that are often not traditional partners: environmental citizen groups and manufacturers, health professionals and churches, employers and hospitals. Important to the success of these partnerships are information networks and coordinating mechanisms, both of which can help streamline services and interventions.

Schools offer a natural locus for the provision of crosscutting educational interventions in health, and studies have shown that school health education is an effective means of helping children improve their health knowledge and develop attitudes that facilitate healthier behaviors. Yet only 25 States currently mandate comprehensive school health education programs, and implementation is spotty in even these States.

Similarly, the workplace can be an excellent site for health promotion programs. More than 85 percent of adult Americans spend much of their day at their workplace. Numerous studies have shown the benefits of worksite health promotion programs in improving employee health, reducing insurance claims, improving morale, reducing absenteeism, and reducing employee turnover. Among workplaces with more than 50 employees, about two-thirds report offering at least one health promotion activity.[71] A much smaller share offers a comprehensive package to employees, and even fewer include special activities for family members or retirees.

To enhance educational and community-based programs, by the year 2000...

8.4   **Provide quality K-12 school health education in at least 75% of schools**

8.6   **Provide employee health promotion activities in at least 85% of workplaces with 50 or more employees**
(a 31% increase)

Other objectives target increasing reading levels and high school graduation rates; increasing preschool programs for disadvantaged children; strengthening the public health system; increasing accessibility of health promotion programs for older people; development of broad State-based strategies for health promotion; and stronger focus on the health promotion needs of minorities.

Health Protection

Unintentional Injuries

Occupational Safety and Health

Environmental Health

Food and Drug Safety

Oral Health

Unintentional Injuries

Unintentional injuries are the fourth leading cause of death in the United States, killing about 100,000 people a year, and are a major cause of disability.[51] Nonfatal injuries are responsible for one of every six hospital days and one of every 10 hospital discharges.[81] Nearly two-thirds of all injury deaths and 84 percent of all injuries resulting in hospitalization involve unintentional injuries. Motor vehicle crashes account for approximately one-half of the deaths from unintentional injuries. Deaths from falls rank second, followed by deaths from poisoning, drowning, and residential fires.[17]

At highest risk are the young and older adults. During the first four decades of life injuries account for more deaths than either chronic or infectious diseases, taking more than 2 million potential years of life from Americans every year. Males are more than twice as likely to die from unintentional injuries than females, and blacks have higher death rates than whites.[51] American Indian and Alaska Natives have disproportionately higher injury death rates.[30]

Injuries have been estimated to cost the United States more than $100 billion annually due to lost productivity and medical care, with a third of these costs attributable to falls and 28 percent to motor vehicle crashes.[81]

About 46,000 people die and 3,500,000 people are injured annually in motor vehicle crashes. By themselves, motor vehicle crashes rank as the fifth leading cause of death in the United States, and approximately half of these are alcohol-related. Alcohol-related traffic crashes are the leading cause of death and spinal cord injury for young Americans.[60]

Although use of automobile safety restraints has increased in recent years, only 42 percent of people currently report using them. Increasing this share to 85 percent could save about 10,000 lives per year. Given the fact that almost 30 percent of motor vehicle fatalities are related to motorcycle, pedestrian, and bicycle casualities, increasing helmet use could also prove of substantial benefit.[61,62]

Many injuries are multifactorial in nature. Alcohol use is a factor in numerous unintentional injuries, including about half of all motor vehicle fatalities and a sizable share of drownings. Of the 33,000 firearm-related deaths in 1987, nearly 3,400 were children aged 1 through 19.[14] Of these, about 15 percent were unintentional and often due to improper handling, accessibility to children, and lack of safety mechanisms.[14] Progress in reducing unintentional injuries will require full participation of the fields of education, transportation, law, engineering, architecture, and safety sciences.

To reduce unintentional injuries, by the year 2000...

**9.1   Reduce unintentional injury deaths to no more than 29.3 per 100,000 people
(a 15% decrease)**

**9.12   Increase automobile safety restraint use to at least 85% of occupants
(a 102% increase)**

Other objectives target death from motor vehicle crashes, falls, drownings, and residential fires; occurrence of hip fractures, poisonings, head injuries, and spinal cord injuries; use of protective helmets; extension of safety belt and motorcycle helmet use laws; handgun design; expanded installation of fire sprinklers and smoke detectors; better roadway design and markers; injury prevention instruction in schools; and involvement of primary care providers in counseling on safety.

Occupational Safety and Health

Approximately 110 million people make up the American workforce, with most spending major portions of their days in their work environments. Of the estimated 10 million injuries that occur annually among workers, about 3 million are severe and include some 3,400 to 11,000 deaths. Although the number of fatal occupational injuries has gradually declined in recent years, work-related illnesses and nonfatal injuries appear to be increasing. During 1987, permanent impairments suffered on the job grew from 60,000 to 70,000, total disabling injuries numbered 1.8 million, and combined occupational illnesses and injuries in the manufacturing industries increased by 12 percent.[7]

Approximately 40 percent of work-related fatalities involved people between 25 and 44 years old. More than 20 percent of fatal occupational injuries in the mid-1980s involved highway vehicles, which were the leading cause of death in seven of eight industry divisions. Other causes included falls (13 percent), nonhighway industrial vehicular injuries (11 percent), blows other than by vehicles or equipment (8 percent), and electrocutions (7 percent). Other leading work-related problems include occupational lung diseases, musculoskeletal injuries, and occupational cancers.[7]

Those occupations with relatively higher rates of injury include mining, agriculture, construction, manufacturing, trucking, and warehousing. The largest numbers (as opposed to rates) of injuries occur in industries with large total workforces such as eating and drinking establishments, grocery stores, hospitals, trucking companies, nursing homes, department stores, and hotels/motels. While employees in occupations related to these enterprises comprise about one-fifth of the total workforce, they report one-fourth of the injuries.[7]

Prevention of occupational health hazards rests on the basic principles of control technology: engineering controls, work practices, personal protective equipment, and monitoring of the workplace for emerging hazards. Despite the number of occupational injuries, effective prevention is practiced in many workplaces, and approximately 48 percent of all establishments report no injuries in a given year.

To improve occupational safety and health, by the year 2000...

10.1 Reduce work-related injury deaths to no more than 4 per 100,000 workers (a 33% decrease)

10.2 Reduce work-related injuries to no more than 6 per 100 workers (a 22% decrease)

Other objectives target reductions in cumulative trauma disorders (e.g., from repetitive motion, pressure, or noise), occupational skin disorders, and, among health workers, hepatitis B infection; use of occupant protection systems by workers; reducing workplace exposure to lead; State implementation of plans for identification and control of major work-related illnesses and injuries; State standards to prevent work-related lung disease; increasing worksites with formal plans for worker health and safety, including back injury prevention programs; expanded State assistance to small businesses in implementation of worker health and safety programs; and greater attention by primary health care providers to occupational health exposures.

Environmental Health

Environmental measures have long been a mainstay of public health. State and local efforts to assure safe supplies of food and water, to manage sewage and municipal wastes, and to control or eliminate vector-borne illnesses have contributed substantially to public health improvements in the United States. The most difficult challenges for environmental health today come from uncertainties about the toxic and ecologic effects of the use of fossil fuels and synthetic chemicals in modern society. An estimated 82 percent of major industrial chemicals have not been tested for their toxic properties and links to specific diseases, and only a small proportion of chemicals have been adequately tested for their ability to cause or promote cancer.[68] Still, enough is known to target improvement in several areas.

Exposure to lead, air pollutants, and radon are good examples. Exposure to high levels of lead is toxic to the central nervous system and can be fatal. Even low levels of exposure can result in persistent impairments in central nervous system function, especially in children, including delayed learning, impaired hearing, and growth deficits. Yet an estimated 2 out of 3 poor inner-city black children aged 6 months through 5 years have blood lead levels above 15 µg/dL and 1 out of 10 has levels above 25 µg/dL. For the Nation as a whole, nearly 3 million children are at some risk from elevated lead levels.[1] Decreased levels of lead in gasoline, air, and food and releases from industrial sources have resulted in lower mean blood lead levels. However, lead in paint, dust, and soil in inner-city urban areas has been lowered only to a limited extent. A strong national effort is needed to reduce lead in the home environment.

Airborne pollutants have been shown to contribute to lung diseases, bronchial asthma, cancer, neural disorders, and eye irritation.[21] Standards have been set by the Environmental Protection Agency for ozone, carbon monoxide, particulates, sulfur dioxide, nitrogen dioxide, and lead. Air quality has improved greatly since 1970, but in 1988 less than 50 percent of Americans lived in counties that met all the EPA standards for air quality for the previous 12 months.[22] Additional measures are necessary to reduce contamination from motor vehicles and other sources.

Radon comes from rock and soil, enters buildings through cracks in foundations or basements, and when inhaled releases ionizing radiation that can damage lung tissue and lead to lung cancer. Along with tobacco smoke, it is a leading indoor air hazard, and as many as an estimated 8 million homes may have radon at a level requiring correction.[21] Low-cost test kits are available to identify exposures, but only about 5 percent of homes have been tested.[72]

To improve environmental health, by the year 2000...

11.4 **Eliminate blood lead levels above 25 µg/dL in children under age 5**

11.5 **Increase protection from air pollutants so that at least 85% of people live in counties that meet EPA standards**
(a 71% increase)

11.6 **Increase protection from radon so that at least 40% of people live in homes tested by homeowners and found to be/made safe**
(a 700% increase)

Other objectives target reducing infectious agent and chemical contamination of drinking water supplies and surface water; reducing human exposure to toxic agents released into the air, water, and soil; reducing environmental burden of solid waste contamination; eliminating immediate risks from hazardous waste sites; improving household management of recyclable materials and toxic waste materials; and better State-based systems to track environmental exposures and diseases.

Food and Drug Safety

American consumers currently benefit from extensive food and drug safety assurance systems. Microbial contamination of food in the production process is rare. Inspections of foods for pesticide residues consistently find that between 96 and 98 percent of foods tested do not contain pesticides in excess of legal limits—and those limits are typically set with a wide margin for error, 100 to 1,000 times lower than a level causing toxic effects in animals.[23] Similarly, careful procedures are established to test new drugs, and each year FDA officials inspect one-third of 18,000 drug and biologics establishments in the United States to ensure proper manufacture and handling.[24]

Nevertheless, outbreaks of foodborne disease and incidents involving drugs continue to occur and cause illness or death. Some problems are caused by failures in the protective systems established at the Federal, State, and local levels. In many cases, problems are caused by foods improperly handled by consumers, the misuse of a prescribed drug, and drug interactions that occur when different health care providers unknowingly prescribe different drugs for the same patient.

Based on the number and severity of cases that occur, *Salmonella*, *Campylobacter*, *Escherichia coli*, and *Listeria* are four of the most important foodborne pathogens in the United States—largely related to time and temperature abuse of foods. One problem that has increased markedly over the decade of the 1980s is illness due to infection with *Salmonella enteritidis*. This foodborne disease is often traced to contaminated eggs and results in severe diarrhea, fever, vomiting, and can even cause death. The 77 outbreaks occurring in 1989 involved nearly 2,400 cases and 14 deaths.[14] Expanded efforts are needed both to reduce source exposure (e.g., sale of contaminated eggs) and to improve food preparation and handling techniques that can protect against this problem.

The principal drug safety issue of the coming years is related to polypharmacy, the use of multiple prescription and over-the-counter medications, especially by older people with chronic health problems. This problem calls for a coordinated prevention approach, involving care on the part of those who prescribe medications to ensure that they will not adversely interact with previously prescribed drug regimens still in use; attentiveness on the part of pharmacists to spot potential medication problems as their customers purchase new prescription drugs; and education for consumers to help them comply with prescribed pharmacologic therapies.

To ensure food and drug safety, by the year 2000...

12.2   Reduce salmonella infection outbreaks to fewer than 25 yearly (a 68% decrease)

Other objectives target reductions in the incidences of foodborne diseases; improving food handling techniques on the part of consumers; better pharmacy-based systems to provide alerts to customers of potential adverse drug interactions; and more regular review by primary care providers of all medications used by their older patients.

Oral Health

Although the prevalence of dental caries or cavities among children has declined steadily since the 1940s, oral diseases remain a prevalent health problem in the United States. On average, among adults 40 through 44, about 1 out of 4 tooth surfaces have been affected by decay.[66] Currently 53 percent of children aged 6 to 8 and 78 percent of 15 year olds have caries.[67] Tooth loss is a major problem among people aged 65 and older, with nearly 40 percent of those aged 65 and older having no natural teeth in 1986.[53] Periodontal diseases, especially gingivitis, also affect many adults. The total cost of dental care to the Nation was more than $27 billion in 1988.[28]

Regular care is a factor in maintaining oral health. However, nearly half the population in the United States does not obtain regular oral health care, and among low-income people the proportion not receiving care is higher.[53] The proportions of black and Hispanic adolescents with untreated decay are approximately 65 percent higher than for the total population.[57,67] One out of every four American Indian and Alaska Native adults aged 35 through 44, and nearly three out of four aged 55 and older, has fewer than 20 natural teeth.

Among preventive measures, community water fluoridation is the single most effective and efficient means of preventing dental caries in children and adults, regardless of race or income level. Yet more than one-third of people with community water systems do not have adequate fluoride, and only about half of those without fluoridated water receive fluoride from other sources.[10] Improvements are needed. Other factors that can improve oral health include regular self-care, avoiding foods that promote caries, and not using tobacco. Excessive alcohol consumption also affects oral health.

Oral cancer is also a serious problem, with 30,000 new cases and 8,600 deaths a year.[88] In fact, oral cancer deaths are more numerous than deaths from cervical cancer. Because 75 percent of oral cancers can be attributed to tobacco and alcohol use, they are preventable. Moreover, because early treatment can reduce mortality, attention is needed for its early detection.

To improve oral health, by the year 2000...

13.1 **Reduce the prevalence of dental caries to no more than 35% of children by age 8**
(a 34% decrease)

13.4 **Reduce edentulism to no more than 20 percent in people aged 65 and older**
(a 44% decrease)

Other objectives target expanding treatment of dental caries; reducing periodontal disease and tooth loss; increasing use of protective sealants on permanent teeth in children; improving parental practices that prevent baby bottle tooth decay; and improving use of oral health screening and follow-up services for all age groups.

Preventive Services

Maternal and Infant Health

Heart Disease and Stroke

Cancer

Diabetes and Chronic Disabling Conditions

HIV Infection

Sexually Transmitted Diseases

Immunization and Infectious Diseases

Clinical Preventive Services

Maternal and Infant Health

Of every 1,000 babies born in the United States each year, about 10 die before they reach their first birthday.[70] Although the infant mortality rate in the United States is declining and has reached an all-time low, the pace of progress has slowed. Mortality is also higher for black infants, who die at twice the rate of white infants, and data from the National Birth Cohort Study of 1983 indicate that other minorities may have higher rates than had been estimated previously. Leading causes of deaths among infants are congenital anomalies, sudden infant death syndrome (SIDS), respiratory distress syndrome, and disorders relating to short gestation.[49]

The most prominent risk factor for infant death, low birth weight (less than 2,500 grams), occurred among nearly 7 percent of all births in 1987 and was associated with more than half of all infant deaths. Black babies have twice the risk of having low birth weight. Low birth weight is also linked to a variety of nonfatal disorders, including neurodevelopmental conditions, learning and behavior problems, and lower respiratory tract infections. In 1985, approximately 11,000 low-birth-weight infants were born with moderate to severe disabilities.[55] From 1970 to 1981 low birth weight declined about 1.3 percent per year, but has since been stagnant.[70] A number of risk factors have been identified for low birth weight, including: younger and older maternal age, high parity, poor reproductive history (especially history of low birth weight), low socioeconomic status, low level of education, late entry into prenatal care, low pregnancy weight gain, smoking, and other substance abuse.[35] Smoking is estimated to be associated with from 20 to 30 percent of all low-birth-weight births in this country.[36] Illicit drug use as a contributor to low birth weight has increased in some urban areas.

An expectant mother with no prenatal care is three times more likely to have a low-birth-weight baby. Despite the importance of early prenatal care in protecting against low birth weight and infant deaths, nearly one of every four pregnant women in the United States receives no care in the first trimester of her pregnancy.[70] A disproportionate share of these mothers has low income, less than a high school education, or is very young.[86] Between 1970 and 1980 there was a significant trend toward increasing early entry into prenatal care, but that trend has since plateaued.[70] Contributing to this problem is the fact that an estimated 14 million women of reproductive age have no insurance to cover maternity care.[2]

To improve maternal and infant health, by the year 2000...

14.1 **Reduce infant mortality to no more than 7 deaths per 1,000 births (a 31% decrease)**

14.5 **Reduce low birth weight to no more than 5% of live births (a 28% decrease)**

14.11 **Increase first trimester prenatal care to at least 90% of live births (an 18% increase)**

Other objectives target reducing rates of fetal death, maternal mortality, and fetal alcohol syndrome; increasing abstinence from tobacco, alcohol, cocaine, and marijuana during pregnancy; increasing the proportion of mothers who gain enough weight during their pregnancies, as well as increasing the number who breastfeed their babies; reducing severe complications of pregnancy and cesarean delivery rates; increasing the availability of preconception care and counseling, as well as of genetic services and counseling; improving the management of high risk cases; and increasing the proportion of babies who receive recommended primary care services.

Heart Disease and Stroke

Despite dramatic declines in mortality from heart disease and stroke in the past two decades, about 7 million Americans are affected by coronary artery disease, and cardiovascular diseases still cause more deaths in the United States than all other diseases combined.[51] Reductions in major risk factors—high blood pressure, high blood cholesterol, and smoking—are having a significant impact on cardiovascular mortality.

Approximately 30 percent of adults in America have high blood pressure.[58] People with uncontrolled high blood pressure are at 3 to 4 times the risk of developing coronary heart disease and as much as 7 times the risk of developing a stroke as do those with normal blood pressures.[18] Overall, blacks have a higher prevalence of high blood pressure than whites (38 percent versus 29 percent).[58] Although surveys indicate that most adults with high blood pressure are aware of their condition, only about one-quarter to a third have their blood pressure under control.[57] This remains a problem despite the fact that many can reduce their blood pressure to normal through programs of physical activity and weight loss, reduced sodium and alcohol intake, and stress management; and medications are available for those who cannot.

The National Heart, Lung, and Blood Institute regards a blood cholesterol level below 200 mg/dL as desirable.[58] Yet the mean cholesterol level for Americans is 213 mg/dL,[54] and about 60 million adults in this country are estimated to have blood cholesterol levels that place them at high risk for coronary heart disease.[84] The Coronary Primary Prevention Trial showed that men at high risk were able to reduce coronary heart disease by about 2 percent for every 1 percent lower blood cholesterol level.[40] Most people can lower their high blood cholesterol by reducing their intake of saturated fat, total fat, and dietary cholesterol, and by normalizing their weight and increasing physical activity. Medications are available for those whose blood cholesterol levels remain significantly elevated despite diet modification.

Tobacco use, which may account for as much as 40 percent of heart disease deaths among people under age 65, is discussed elsewhere. Other contributors to cardiovascular disease include obesity, physical inactivity, and diabetes mellitus.

To reduce heart disease and stroke, by the year 2000...

15.1   Reduce coronary heart disease deaths to no more than 100 per 100,000 people
(a 26% decrease)

15.2   Reduce stroke deaths to no more than 20 per 100,000 people
(a 34% decrease)

15.4   Increase control of high blood pressure to at least 50% of people with HBP
(a 108% increase)

15.6   Reduce blood cholesterol to an average of no more than 200 mg/dL
(a 6% decrease)

Other objectives target appropriate management behaviors by those with high blood cholesterol and high blood pressure; reducing dietary fat intake; reducing overweight and increasing physical activity; reducing tobacco use; increasing numbers of adults who have recently been screened for high blood pressure or high blood cholesterol; better use of worksites for detection and followup programs; and improving adherence to recommended protocols and standards for primary care providers and laboratories involved in cholesterol testing and management.

Cancer

Cancer accounts for about one of every five deaths in the United States each year.[3] About 75 million Americans now living, nearly one in three, will eventually have cancer. While the incidence of cancer has increased in the past two decades, death rates for those under 55 have fallen.[47] More people are surviving cancer now than several decades ago. Not everyone, however, has benefitted equally from this trend. Blacks are less likely than whites to survive 5 years from the time of diagnosis. The five-year survival rate for all cancer sites combined is 50 percent for white patients and 37 percent for black patients.

Once surrounded by fear and fatalism, cancer has been the focus of nationwide educational campaigns to inform the public that the risk of cancer can be significantly reduced when adequate preventive measures are taken. Tobacco has been estimated to account for 30 percent of cancers, and dietary factors roughly another 35 percent.[48] For example, most cases of lung cancer, the leading cause of cancer mortality, can be prevented by not smoking, and epidemiological research suggests that diets relatively low in fat and higher in foods containing fiber may help prevent colon, rectal, breast, prostate, and other cancers. High levels of alcohol use have been linked to esophageal and oral cancers. Limiting sun exposure, use of sunscreens and protective clothing when exposed to sunlight, and avoidance of sun lamps and tanning booths can reduce the risk of skin cancer.

Early detection also can have an important impact on cancer death rates. Procedures such as mammography and clinical breast examination, the Pap test, fecal occult blood tests, proctosigmoidoscopy, and oral, skin, and digital rectal examinations make it possible to treat cancers before they spread. For example, research suggests than breast cancer deaths could be reduced by 30 percent among women aged 50 and older through the use of mammography and clinical breast examination.[85,89,93] Yet in 1987, only 25 percent of such women had these tests within the preceding 2 years. A Pap test could reduce cervical cancer deaths by an estimated 75 percent, but one out of every five women with family incomes less than $10,000 has never had a Pap test.[53] Despite the fact that fecal occult blood testing and sigmoidoscopy are important to facilitate early diagnosis of colorectal cancer, especially among those at high risk, only 27 percent of people aged 50 and older report receiving a fecal occult blood test within the preceding 2 years.

To prevent and control cancer, by the year 2000...

16.1   Reverse the rise in cancer deaths to no more than 130 per 100,000 people

**16.11   Increase clinical breast exams and mammography every 2 years to at least 60% of women aged 50 and older
(a 140% increase)**

**16.12   Increase Pap tests every 1-3 years to at least 85% of women aged 18 and older
(a 13% increase)**

**16.13   Increase fecal occult blood testing every 1-2 years to at least 50% of people aged 50 and older
(an 85% increase)**

Other objectives target reducing dietary fat intake; increasing consumption of vegetables, fruits, and grain products; reducing tobacco use; decreasing sun exposure; more counseling by primary care providers on diet and tobacco use and offering of screening procedures according to established protocols; and improving the quality of Pap tests and mammograms.

Diabetes and Chronic Disabling Conditions

As the population of the United States grows older, the problems posed by chronic and disabling conditions increasingly demand the Nation's attention. Chronic conditions such as heart disease, cancer, stroke, and lung and liver disease are joined in importance by other chronic and disabling conditions, affecting people in all age groups, such as diabetes, arthritis, deformities or orthopedic impairments, hearing and speech impairments, and mental retardation.

Chronic and disabling conditions have a profound effect not only on mortality rates but also on quality of life. Disability, defined by its impact on major activities one is able to perform, affected more than 9 percent of Americans in 1988.[50] About 33 million people have functional limitations that interfere with their daily activities, and more than 9 million have limitations that prevent them from working, attending school, or maintaining a household. The underlying impairments most often responsible for these conditions are arthritis, heart disease, back conditions (including spinal curvature), lower extremity impairments, and intervertebral disk disorders.[37] For those under age 18 the most frequent causes of activity limitation are asthma, mental retardation, mental illness, and hearing and speech impairments.

Diabetes is one of the most prevalent chronic conditions among Americans. Approximately 7 million people in the United States have been diagnosed with diabetes and each year some 650,000 new cases are identified. In 1987, diabetes was the underlying cause of death for more than 37,000 Americans and contributed to over 100,000 additional deaths. According to the American Diabetes Association, in addition to death, diabetes is accountable for 30 percent of kidney failure cases, is the second leading cause of blindness in people aged 45 through 74, causes half of all nontraumatic amputations, and causes a threefold increase in risk for congenital malformations and perinatal mortality among babies of diabetic mothers. Insulin-dependent diabetes mellitus (IDDM or Type I) is the most severe form, but comprises no more than 10 percent of all cases of diabetes. Noninsulin-dependent diabetes mellitus (NIDDM or Type II), while serious, has less severe consequences, usually appears after age 40, is often associated with obesity, and may often be controlled by diet and exercise, sometimes in combination with oral hypoglycemic agents. Careful control of diabetes is critical to prevention of its complications. Diet and physical activity are important to the management of both types of diabetes, and NIDDM can often be prevented through these measures.

To reduce diabetes and chronic disabling conditions, by the year 2000...

17.2 Reduce disability from chronic conditions to no more than 8% of people (a 15% decrease)

17.9 Reduce diabetes-related deaths to no more than 34 per 100,000 people (an 11% decrease)

Other objectives target reducing reducing complications of diabetes; reducing disability from asthma, chronic back conditions, osteoporosis, hearing impairment, vision impairment, and mental retardation; increasing physical activity; reducing overweight; improving early diagnosis and referral for disabling conditions among the very young and older people; improving community and self-help resources for people with chronic and disabling conditions; and improving employer policies related to the needs of people with disabilities.

HIV Infection

The human immunodeficiency virus (HIV) epidemic is a multifaceted national and international problem. People with HIV infection can develop acquired immunodeficiency syndrome (AIDS), including severe opportunistic infections, Kaposi's sarcoma, and multiple-system medical complications. Without treatment about 50 percent of people develop AIDS within 10 years of becoming infected with HIV, and another 40 percent or more develop other clinical illnesses associated with HIV infection.[29] By the end of 1989, reported cases of AIDS had reached 115,000,[12] but the projected figure is expected to more than triple or quadruple by the end of 1993. It has become the seventh leading cause of potential years of life lost in the United States. By the end of 1993, a projected total of 390,000 to 480,000 cases of AIDS will have been diagnosed in the United States and 285,000 to 340,000 people will have died from the disease.[14] Annual costs of AIDS are projected to climb as high as $5 to $13 billion by 1992.[14,43]

An estimated 1 million people in the United States are infected with HIV and of these approximately 40,000 became infected in 1989. Groups at special risk have been identified and include: intravenous drug abusers and their sex partners; people with large numbers of sex partners; men who have sex with men, and their female partners; and people who exchange sex for money or drugs. Of current AIDS patients, more than three-fourths are male, and two-thirds are male homosexuals and bisexuals; but the most rapid increases are occurring among intravenous drug-abusers, women, and babies born to women in high risk groups. An estimated 20 to 35 percent of infants of infected mothers develop HIV infection. Approximately 60 percent of AIDS patients are white, 25 percent are black, and 15 percent are Hispanic.[12]

Although some therapeutic agents may extend survival, there is currently no available treatment to prevent death among people with AIDS. The survival rate in the early 1980s was only about 15 percent, before the licensure of antiviral drugs, such as zidovudine (AZT). AZT has been shown to slow replication of the virus and improve survival prospects, as have selected other agents now under study.

The development of a safe and effective HIV vaccine is a high priority for the coming decade, although the prospects for the availability of such a vaccine are uncertain. Other prevention and control strategies are vital to stopping the spread of HIV infection. Most HIV-infected people in the United States do not know they harbor the virus, and increased counseling, testing, and follow-up services are needed. Public education efforts on risks and precautions are essential to slowing the spread of the disease.

To prevent and control HIV infection, by the year 2000...

18.2 Confine HIV infection to no more than 800 per 100,000 people

Other objectives target reducing experience with sexual intercourse among adolescents; increasing use of condoms among sexually active, unmarried people; increasing outreach and access to treatment programs for intravenous drug abusers; expanding testing and counseling for people at risk of HIV infection, including improved skills among primary care providers; increasing education in schools and colleges about HIV infection and its prevention; and extension of regulations to protect workers at risk for occupational transmission of HIV.

Sexually Transmitted Diseases

Sexually transmitted diseases affect almost 12 million Americans each year, 86 percent of whom are aged 15 through 29.[11] About one-fifth of all young people, by the time they reach 21, have needed treatment for a sexually transmitted disease.[94] Because only some teenagers are sexually active, this amounts to an effective rate of at least 25 percent among those who are. The sexually transmitted diseases encompass more than 50 recognized organisms and syndromes, including, in addition to syphilis and gonorrhea, *chlamydia trachomatis* infections, genital herpes, hepatitis B, chancroid, cytomegalovirus, and human immunodeficiency virus (HIV). After AIDS, the most serious complications of sexually transmitted diseases are pelvic inflammatory disease (PID), sterility, ectopic pregnancy, blindness, cancer associated with human papillomavirus, fetal and infant death, birth defects, and mental retardation. The total societal cost of sexually transmitted diseases exceeds $3.5 billion annually, with the cost of PID and PID-associated ectopic pregnancy and infertility alone exceeding $2.6 billion.[94]

Gonorrhea is the most frequently reported communicable disease in the United States. In 1989, some 733,000 cases were reported and the incidence was an estimated 300 per 100,000 people. Youth, low-income, and minority populations are at particular risk. In 1989, adolescents aged 15 through 19 had an infection rate of 1,125 per 100,000 and blacks a rate of 1,990 per 100,000. Despite the fact that since 1981, cases of gonorrhea in males have declined 29 percent and declined 24 percent in females, the rates have not declined among racial and ethnic minorities or among teenagers. Furthermore, the percent of all gonorrhea organisms that are antibiotic-resistant grew from less than 1 percent in 1985 to 7 percent in 1989.[10]

In 1989, nearly 45,000 cases of syphilis were also reported. Syphilis is the first sexually transmitted disease for which control measures were developed and tested. Since the initiation of Federal assistance for syphilis control in the 1940s, reported cases of all stages of syphilis declined from an all-time high of 575,600 cases in 1943 to fewer than 68,000 cases in 1985. In recent years, however, the number of syphilis cases has increased dramatically, due in part to an increase in the exchange of sex for drugs, to an increased number of crack cocaine users, and to increased sexual activity among adolescents. Between 1986 and 1989, the number of reported syphilis cases increased over 55 percent, to the highest level in the United States since the early 1950s.[10]

To reduce sexually transmitted diseases, by the year 2000...

**19.1   Reduce gonorrhea infections to no more than 225 per 100,000 people
(a 25% decrease)**

**19.3   Reduce syphilis infections to no more than 10 per 100,000 people
(a 45% decrease)**

Other objectives target reducing infections with *chlamydia trachomatis*, genital herpes and genital warts, and hepatitis B; reducing occurrence of pelvic inflammatory disease; increasing use of condoms among sexually active, unmarried people; fuller availability of comprehensive sexually transmitted disease-related services in clinics and centers that provide family planning, maternal and child health care, drug treatment, and primary care to low income families; increasing partner tracing and notification; improving primary care provider management of STD cases; and inclusion of instruction on STD transmission and prevention as part of school health education for middle and secondary school students.

Immunization and Infectious Diseases

The reduction in incidence of infectious diseases is the most significant public health achievement of the past 100 years. This success is most notably embodied in the global eradication of smallpox, achieved in 1977. Other gains in control of infectious diseases are nearly as striking, including the virtual elimination of diphtheria and poliomyelitis in the United States. Much of the progress made has been a result of improvements in basic hygiene, food production and food handling, and water treatment. The development and use of antimicrobial drugs have reduced the morbidity and mortality associated with a number of infectious diseases. The other major factor in reducing the toll from infectious diseases has been the development and widespread use of vaccines, which are among the safest and most effective measures for the prevention of infectious diseases.

Nevertheless, infectious diseases still cause many preventable illnesses and deaths. Influenza and pneumonia, for example, shorten the lives of many older adults despite the availability of vaccines. Approximately 80 to 90 percent of all influenza-associated deaths in the United States occur in people 65 years or older.[9] The childhood vaccine-preventable diseases, although they have declined dramatically, remain problems among certain high-risk, under-immunized groups. Moreover, newly recognized diseases, such as Legionnaire's disease, toxic shock syndrome, Lyme disease, and the wide spectrum of diseases associated with human immunodeficiency virus infection, have emerged as threats to public health.

The occurrence of measles in the United States is an example of an infectious disease problem that should be readily controlled in that a vaccine has been available since 1963. Use of that vaccine helped to reduce the number of reported measles cases in this country to an all-time-low of under 1,500 in 1983. However, due to inadequate immunization of low-income preschool children, as well as of young people, the disease has demonstrated a resurgence in susceptible populations, with over 16,000 cases reported in 1989, including 41 deaths.[42] In response, the measles immunization protocol recommended by the Immunization Practices Advisory Committee now calls for a two-dose schedule of measles vaccine, but effective control will also require better outreach in low-income communities, continued strong enforcement of school entry laws, and efficient identification and intervention in disease outbreaks.

To increase immunization and prevent infectious diseases, by the year 2000...

20.1   Eliminate measles

20.2   Reduce epidemic-related pneumonia and influenza deaths to no more than 7.3 per 100,000 people aged 65 and older (a 20% decrease)

20.11 Increase childhood immunization levels to at least 90% of 2 year-olds (a 20% increase)

Other objectives target eliminating indigenous cases of diphtheria, tetanus, polio, and rubella; reducing viral hepatitis, tuberculosis, bacterial meningitis; reducing infectious diarrhea among children in licensed child care centers; reducing middle ear infections; increasing immunization levels for pneumococcal pneumonia and hepatitis B; expanding immunization laws for schools, preschools, and child care settings; eliminating financial barriers to immunizations; fully involving primary care providers in meeting the immunization needs of their patients; and expanding laboratory capabilities for rapid viral diagnosis of influenza.

Clinical Preventive Services

Clinical preventive services refer to those disease prevention and health promotion services—immunizations, screening, and counseling—delivered to individuals in a health care setting. The effectiveness of preventive services in reducing disease, disability, and premature death is now well documented. The dramatic declines observed for childhood infectious diseases and early death from strokes and cervical cancer are largely attributed to the widespread application of three preventive services: childhood immunizations, high blood pressure detection and control, and Pap tests. Several other preventive services, such as screening mammography, have also been shown to be effective. In 1989, the U.S. Preventive Services Task Force reported on its review of the scientific evidence on 169 clinical preventive services for 60 target conditions. Based on well-established criteria, it published in the *Guide to Clinical Preventive Services*[92] its recommendations on the basic services that should be provided.

Despite their proven effectiveness, clinical preventive services are rarely covered under health insurance or delivered as recommended. The few studies that have examined the receipt of clinical preventive services have found the delivery to be less than optimal. For example, although 93 percent of newborns studied had received at least one well-child examination, less than half had received three or more doses of diphtheria-pertussis-tetanus (DPT) vaccine and three or more doses of polio vaccine by age 18 months.[41] The National Health Interview Survey found an increase in the use of eight routine preventive services among adults and children between 1973 and 1982, but low-income people, people with low levels of education, and people of Hispanic origin were among the least likely to have ever received all eight procedures.[19] A related study found that only 42 percent of women had adequately received a blood pressure check, clinical breast examination, Pap test, and glaucoma screening.[96] Screening was less adequate among the poor, the less educated, and those living in rural areas, with only 33, 34, and 38 percent, respectively, screened for all four conditions.

Barriers specific to the delivery or use of preventive services include uncertainty among health care providers about which services to offer, practice organization characteristics that are not conducive to delivery of preventive services (e.g., lack of time, too few allied health professionals, and limited access to medical record systems organized for prevention), and inadequate knowledge among consumers to create the necessary demand. Another important barrier is the lack of reimbursement or financing. In addition to the fact that few insurance plans cover preventive services, a substantial proportion of Americans—some 30 to 37 million—are without any form of health insurance. And many more are underinsured or are covered by insurance programs with requirements and payments that providers are increasingly reluctant to accept.

To expand access and use of clinical preventive services, by the year 2000...

21.4 Eliminate financial barriers to clinical preventive services

Other objectives target increasing the proportion of people with a specific source of ongoing primary care; increasing primary care providers' delivery of recommended preventive services; increasing the number of people who receive recommended clinical preventive services; increasing delivery of preventive services to patients of publicly funded providers of primary care; and increasing representation of minorities among primary care providers.

Surveillance and Data Systems

Surveillance and Data Systems

Systematically collecting, analyzing, interpreting, disseminating, and using health data is essential to understanding the health status of a population and to planning effective prevention programs. Public health surveillance and data systems collect information on morbidity, mortality, disability, injuries, risk factors, services, and costs. Systems used in the United States include vital statistics and disease reporting systems as well as sample surveys, such as the continuous National Health Interview Survey (NHIS).

Although the United States Public Health Service takes the lead role in national public health data collection, it is only one partner within the larger structure necessary to collect national public health data. Surveillance often requires active cooperation among Federal, State, and local agencies. For example, the National Vital Statistics System obtains information on births, deaths, marriages, and divorces from all 50 States, New York City, the District of Columbia, Puerto Rico, the United States Virgin Islands, and Guam. Programs in each State collect vital information from many sources in local communities, including funeral directors, medical examiners, coroners, hospitals, religious authorities, and justices of the peace. Other surveys, like the National Health Interview Survey, are based on interviews with thousands of individual citizens nationwide. Still others, like the Centers for Disease Control's Behavioral Risk Factor Surveillance System, are based on State reports of telephone interviews with individual citizens.

The Institute of Medicine's report, *The Future of Public Health*, recognized the importance of surveillance and data systems for guiding public health into the 21st century, in recommending the creation and use of methods for the collection of "...national data that will permit comparison of local and State health data with those of the Nation and of other States and localities and that will facilitate progress towards the national health objectives..."[31] The development and dissemination of comparable procedures for data collection would facilitate comparability of data on health status within and among State and local areas and would permit the valid comparison of local and State health data with national data. In addition, the development of a small set of common health indicators, arrived at through a consensus process, would facilitate communication among public health officials and with others involved in programs and activities that affect the Nation's health (e.g., employers and school administrators). Though complete comparability across data systems is not possible given the differences in purposes and approaches (e.g., direct interviews v. telephone v. mail), differences can be minimized.

To improve surveillance and data systems, by the year 2000...

22.1 Develop and implement common health status indicators for use by Federal/State/local health agencies

Other objectives target creation of data sources to track the year 2000 objectives; expanded State-based activity to track the progress of the population toward the year 2000 objectives; improvement of related data for blacks, Hispanics, American Indians and Alaska Natives, Asian Americans, and people with disabilities; improvement of information transfer capabilities among Federal, State, and local agencies; and more speedy processing of survey and surveillance data.

References

1 Agency for Toxic Substances and Disease Registry. *The Nature and Extent of Lead Poisoning in Children in the United States: A Report to Congress.* Washington, DC: U.S. Department of Health and Human Services, July 1988.

2 The Alan Guttmacher Institute. *Blessed Events and the Bottom Line: The Financing of Maternity Care in the United States.* New York: the Institute, 1987.

3 American Cancer Society. *Cancer Facts and Figures - 1989.* New York: the Society, 1990.

4 American School Health Association; Association for the Advancement of Health Education; and Society for Public Health Education, Inc. *The National Adolescent Student Health Survey.* Oakland, CA: the Third Party Publishing Company, 1989.

5 Blair, S.N.; Kohl, H.W.; Paffenbarger, R.S.; Clark, D.G.; Cooper, K.H.; and Gibbons, L.W. Physical fitness and all-cause mortality: A prospective study of healthy men and women. *JAMA* 262:2395-2401, 1989.

6 Boyd, J.H., and Moscicki, E.K.. Firearms and youth suicide. *American Journal of Public Health* 76:1240-1242, 1986.

7 Bureau of Labor Statistics. *Annual Survey of Occupational Injuries and Illnesses.* Washington, DC: Department of Labor, 1988.

8 Cady, L.D.; Bischoff, D.P.; O'Connell, E.R.; Thomas, P.C.; and Allan, J.H. Strength and fitness and subsequent back injuries in firefighters. *Journal of Occupational Medicine* 21:269-272, 1979.

9 Center for Infectious Diseases, Centers for Disease Control, Public Health Service, U.S. Department of Health and Human Services, Atlanta, GA.

10 Center for Prevention Services, Centers for Disease Control, Public Health Service, U.S. Department of Health and Human Services, Atlanta, GA.

11 Centers for Disease Control. *Division of STD/HIV Prevention Annual Report, 1989.* Atlanta, GA: U.S. Department of Health and Human Services, 1990.

12 Centers for Disease Control. *HIV/AIDS Surveillance Report.* Atlanta, GA: U.S. Department of Health and Human Services, May 1990.

13 Centers for Disease Control. *Homicide Surveillance: High-Risk Racial and Ethnic Groups/Blacks and Hispanics, 1970 to 1983.* Atlanta, GA: U.S. Department of Health and Human Services, 1986.

14 Centers for Disease Control, Public Health Service, U.S. Department of Health and Human Services, Atlanta, GA.

15 Centers for Disease Control In: U.S Preventive Services Task Force. *Guide to Clinical Preventive Services: An Assessment of the Effectiveness of 169 Interventions.* Baltimore, MD: Williams and Wilkins, 1989.

16 Centers for Disease Control. Years of potential life lost before age 65: United States, 1987. *MMWR* 38:27-9, 1989.

17 Committee on Trauma Research, Commission on Life Sciences, National Research Council, and Institute of Medicine. *Injury in America: A Continuing Public Health Problem.* Washington, DC: National Academy Press, 1988.

18 Dawber, T.R. *The Framingham Study: The Epidemiology of Atherosclerotic Disease.* Cambridge, MA: Harvard University Press, 1980.

19 Dawson, D.A.; Hendershot, G.E.; Bloom, B. Trends in routine screening examinations. *American Journal of Public Health* 77(8):1004-1005, 1987.

20 Dryfoos, J.G. *Working Paper on Youth At Risk: One in Four in Jeopardy.* Hastings-on-the-Hudson, New York: Report submitted to the Carnegie Corporation, 1987.

21 Environmental Protection Agency. *Environmental Progress and Challenges: EPA's Update.* Washington, DC: U.S. Environmental Protection Agency, August 1988.

22 Environmental Protection Agency. *National Air Quality and Emissions Trends Report, 1988.* EPA-450/4-90-002. Washington, DC: U.S. Environmental Protection Agency, 1990.

23 Farley, D. *Setting Safe Limits on Pesticide Residues, Safety First: Protecting America's Food Supply, a special report of FDA Consumer.* Washington, DC: U.S. Department of Health and Human Services, 1988.

24 Food and Drug Administration. *From Test Tube to Patient: New Drug Development in the United States, an FDA Consumer Special Report.* Washington, DC: U.S. Department of Health and Human Services, 1988.

25 Harlow, C.W. *Injuries from Crime.* Washington, DC: U.S. Department of Justice, 1989.

26 Harris, S.S.; Casperson, C.J.; DeFriese, G.H.; and Estes, E.H. Physical activity counseling for healthy adults as a primary preventive intervention in the clinical setting. *JAMA* 261:3590-3598, 1989.

27 Harwood, H.J.; Napolitana, D.M.; Kristiansen, P.L.; and Collins, J.J. *Economic Costs to Society of Alcohol and Drug Abuse and Mental Illness: 1980.* Research Triangle Park, NC: Research Triangle Institute, 1984.

28 Health Care Financing Administration, data release, 1990.

29 Hessol, N.A.; Rutherford, G.W.; Lifson, A.R.; et al. "The Natural History of HIV Infection in a Cohort of Homosexual and Bisexual Men: A Decade of Follow Up." Abstract 4096. Proceedings of the IV International Conference on AIDS, Stockholm, Sweden, June 14, 1988.

30 Indian Health Service. *Trends in Indian Health, 1989.* Washington, DC: U.S. Department of Health and Human Services, 1989.

31 Institute of Medicine, National Academy of Sciences. *The Future of Public Health.* Washington, DC: National Academy Press, 1988.

32 Jones, E.F.; Forrest, J.D.; Goldman, N; Henshaw, S.; Lincoln, R.; Rosoff, J.I.; Westoff, C.F.; and Wulf, D. *Teenage Pregnancy in Industrialized Countries: A Study Sponsored by the Alan Guttmacher Institute* New Haven, CT: Yale University Press, 1986.

33 Katz, S.; Branch, L.G.; Branson, M.H.; Papsidero, J.A.; Beck, J.C.; and Greer, D.S. Active life expectancy. *New England Journal of Medicine* 309:1218-1224, 1983.

34 Kleinman, J.C.; and Kopstein, A. Smoking during pregnancy 1967-1980. *American Journal of Public Health* 77:823-825, 1987.

35 Kleinman, J.C., and Kessel, S.S. Racial differences in low birthweight: Trends and risk factors. *New England Journal of Medicine* 317:749-753, 1987.

36 Kleinman, J.C., and Madans, J.H. The effects of maternal smoking, physical stature, and educational attainment on the incidence of low birthweight. *American Journal of Epidemiology* 121(6):843-855, 1985.

37 LaPlante, M.P. *Data on Disability from the National Health Interview Survey, 1983-85.* An InfoUse Report. Washington, D.C.: National Institute on Disability and Rehabilitation Research, 1988.

38 Leon, A.S. Effects of physical activity and fitness on health. In: National Center for Health Statistics. *Assessing Physical Fitness and Physical Activity in Population-Based Surveys.* DHHS Pub. No. (PHS)89-1253. Hyattsville, MD: U.S. Department of Health and Human Services, 1989.

39 Leon, A.S.; Connett, J.; Jacobs, D.R.; and Raurama, R. Leisure-time physical activity levels and risk of coronary heart disease and death: The multiple risk factor intervention trial. *JAMA* 258:2388-2395, 1987.

40 Lipid Research Clinics Program. The lipid research clinics coronary primary prevention trial results: I. Reduction in the incidence of coronary heart disease. *JAMA* 251:351-364, 1984.

41 Lurie, N.; Manning, W.G.; Peterson, C.; Goldberg, G.A.; Phelps, C.A.; and Lillard, L. Preventive care: Do we practice what we preach? *American Journal of Public Health* 77:801-804, 1987.

42 Markowitz, L.E., et al. Patterns of transmission in measles outbreaks in the United States, 1985-1986. *New England Journal of Medicine* 320(2):75-81, 1989.

43 Mason, J.O. Public Health Considerations: A Progress Report. Presented at AIDS/Frontline Health Care Conference, 1989.

44 Mercy, J.A., and Houk, V.N. Firearm injuries: A call for science. *New England Journal of Medicine* 319:1283-85, 1988.

45 Monitoring the Future Study (High School Senior Survey), Alcohol, Drug Abuse, and Mental Health Administration, Public Health Service, U.S. Department of Health and Human Services, Rockville, MD.

46 Moscicki, E.K., and Boyd, J.H. Epidemiologic trends in firearm suicides among adolescents. *Pediatrician* 12:52-62, 1985.

47 National Cancer Institute. *1987 Annual Cancer Statistics Review.* DHHS Pub.No. (NIH)88-2789. Bethesda, MD: U.S. Department of Health and Human Services, 1988.

48 National Cancer Institute. Cancer control objectives for the nation: 1985-2000. *National Cancer Institute Monographs* 2 (1986). DHHS Pub. No. (NIH)86-2880. Bethesda, MD: U.S. Department of Health and Human Services, 1986.

49 National Center for Health Statistics. Advance Report of Final Mortality Statistics, 1987. *Monthly Vital Statistics Report.* Vol. 38 No. 5 (Supp.) Hyattsville, MD: U.S. Department of Health and Human Services, 1989.

50 National Center for Health Statistics. Current Estimates from the National Health Interview Survey, United States, 1988. *Vital and Health Statistics.* Series 10, No. 173, DHHS Pub. No. (PHS)89-1501. Hyattsville, MD: U.S. Department of Health and Human Services, 1989.

51 National Center for Health Statistics. *Health, United States, 1989 and Prevention Profile.* DHHS Pub. No. (PHS)90-1232. Washington, DC: U.S. Department of Health and Human Services, 1990.

52 National Center for Health Statistics. *Hispanic Health and Nutrition Examination Survey, 1983-84.* Hyattsville, MD: U.S. Department of Health and Human Services.

53 National Center for Health Statistics. *National Health Interview Survey, 1986.* Hyattsville, MD: U.S. Department of Health and Human Services.

54 National Center for Health Statistics. "Total Serum Cholesterol Levels of Adults 20-74 Years of Age, United States, 1976-80." Data from the National Health Survey, Series II, No. 236. Hyattsville, MD: U.S. Department of Health and Human Services, 1986.

55 National Commission to Prevent Infant Mortality. *Indirect Costs of Infant Mortality and Low Birth Weight.* Washington, DC: the Commission, 1988.

56 National Family Violence Survey 1985, National Institute of Mental Health, Alcohol, Drug Abuse, and Mental Health Administration, Public Health Service, U.S. Department of Health and Human Services, Rockville, MD.

57 National Health and Nutrition Examination Survey, National Center for Health Statistics, Centers for Disease Control, Public Health Service, U.S. Department of Health and Human Services, Hyattsville, MD.

58 National Heart, Lung and Blood Institute. Hypertension prevalence and the status of awareness, treatment, and control in the United States: Final report of the subcommittee on definition and prevalence of the 1984 joint national committee. *Hypertension* 7(3):457-468, 1985.

59 National Heart, Lung, and Blood Institute. *Report of the Expert Panel on Detection, Evaluation, and Treatment of High Blood Cholesterol Adults.* National Cholesterol Education Program. Bethesda, MD: U.S. Department of Health and Human Services, 1988.

60 National Highway Traffic Safety Administration. *The Economic Cost to Society of Motor Vehicle Accidents.* Technical Report DOT HS 809-195, p. 1. Washington, DC: U.S. Department of Transportation, 1987.

61 National Highway Traffic Administration. *The Effectiveness of Motorcycle Helmets in Preventing Fatalities.* Technical Report DOT HS 807-416. Washington, DC: U.S. Department of Transportation, 1989.

62 National Highway Traffic Safety Administration. *Motorcycle Accident Cause Factors and Identification of Countermeasures.* Technical Report DOT HS 805-862. Washington, DC: U.S. Department of Transportation, 1981.

63 National Household Survey of Drug Abuse, National Institute on Drug abuse, Alcohol, Drug Abuse, and Mental Health Administration, Public Health Service, U.S. Department of Health and Human Services, Rockville, MD..

64 National Institute on Alcohol Abuse and Alcoholism. *Seventh Special Report to the U.S. Congress on Alcohol and Health.* Washington, DC: U.S. Department of Health and Human Services, 1988.

65 National Institute on Alcohol Abuse and Alcoholism. *Sixth Special Report to the U.S. Congress on Alcohol and Health.* Washington, DC: U.S. Department of Health and Human Services, 1987.

66 National Institute of Dental Research. *The Oral Health of United States Adults. The National Survey of Oral Health in U.S. Employed Adults and Seniors: 1985-1986.* DHHS Pub. No. (PHS)87-2868. Bethesda, MD: U.S. Department of Health and Human Services, 1987.

67 National Institute of Dental Research. *Oral Health of United States Children. The National Survey of Dental Caries in U.S. School Children, 1986-1987.* DHHS Pub. No. (PHS)89-2247. Bethesda, MD: U.S. Department of Health and Human Services, 1989.

68 National Research Council. *Toxicity Testing: Strategies to Determine Needs and Priorities.* Washington, DC: National Academy Press, 1984.

69 National Survey of Family Growth. National Center for Health Statistics, Centers for Disease Control, Public Health Service, U.S. Department of Health and Human Services, 1988.

70 National Vital Statistics System, National Center for Health Statistics, Centers for Disease Control, Public Health Service, U.S. Department of Health and Human Services, Hyattsville, Maryland.

71 Office of Disease Prevention and Health Promotion. *National Survey of Worksite Health Promotion Activities: A Summary.* Washington, DC: U.S. Department of Health and Human Services, 1987.

72 Office of Radiation Programs, U.S. Environmental Protection Agency, Washington, DC.

73 Office on Smoking and Health. *Reducing the Health Consequences of Smoking: 25 Years of Progress. A Report of the Surgeon General.* DHHS Publication No. (CDC)89-8411. Washington, DC: U.S. Department of Health and Human Services, 1989.

74 Paffenbarger, R.S.; Hyde, R.T.; Wing, A.L.; and Hsieh, C.C. Physical activity, all-cause mortality, and longevity of college alumni. *New England Journal of Medicine* 314:605-613, 1986.

75 Paffenbarger, R.S.; Wing, A.L.; and Hyde, R.T. Physical activity as an index of heart attack risk in college alumni. *American Journal of Epidemiology* 108:161-175, 1978.

76 Perrine, M.; Peck, R.; and Fell, J. Epidemiologic perspectives on drunk driving. In: *Surgeon General's Workshop on Drunk Driving: Background Papers.* Washington, DC: U.S. Department of Health and Human Services, 1988.

77 Powell, K.E.; Caspersen, C.J.; Koplan, J.P.; and Ford, E.S. Physical activity and chronic disease. *American Journal of Clinical Nutrition* 49:999-1006, 1989.

78 Powell, K.E.; Thompson, P.D.; Caspersen, C.J.; and Kendrick, J.S. Physical activity and the incidence of coronary heart disease. *Annual Review of Public Health* 8:253-287, 1987.

79 Public Health Service. *The Surgeon General's Report on Nutrition and Health.* DHHS Pub. No. (PHS)88-50210. Washington, DC: U.S. Department of Health and Human Services, 1988.

80 Rice, D.P.; Kelman, L.S.; Dunmeyer, S. *The Economic Costs of Alcohol and Drug Abuse and Mental Illness.* San Francisco, CA: Institute for Health and Aging, University of California-San Francisco, 1990.

81 Rice, D.P.; MacKenzie, E.J.; Jones, A.S.; Kaufman, S.R.; deLissovoy, G.V.; Max, W.; McLoughlin, E.; Miller, T.R.; Robertson, L.S.; Salkever, D.S.; and Smith, G.S. *Cost of Injury in the United States: A Report to Congress, 1989.* San Francisco, CA: Institute for Health and Aging, University of California and Injury Prevention Center, The Johns Hopkins University, 1989.

82 Sallis, J.F.; Haskell, W.L.; Fortmann, S.P.; Wood, P.D.; and Vranizan, K.M. Moderate-intensity physical activity and cardiovascular risk factors: The Stanford five-city project. *Preventive Medicine* 15:561-568, 1986.

83 Salonen, J.T.; Puska, P.; and Tuomilehto, J. Physical activity and risk of myocardial infarction, cerebral stroke and death: A longitudinal study in Eastern Finland. *American Journal of Epidemiology* 115:526-537, 1982.

84 Sempos, C.; Fulwood, R.; Haines, C.; Carroll, M.; Anda, R.; Williamson, B.F.; Remmington, P.; and Cleeman, J. The Prevalence of High Blood Cholesterol Levels Among Adults in the United States. *JAMA* 262:45-52, 1989.

85 Shapiro, S.; Venet, W.; Strax, L.; and Roeser; R. Selection, Followup, and Analysis in the Health Insurance Plan Study: A Randomized Trial With Breast Cancer Screening. *National Cancer Institute Monographs* 67:65-74, 1985.

86 Singh, S.; Torres, D.; and Forrest, J.D. The need for prenatal care in the United States: Evidence from the 1980 national natality survey. *Family Planning Perspectives* 17:118-124, 1985.

87 Sonnenstein, F.L.; Pleck, J.H.; Ku, L.C. Sexual activity, condom use, and AIDS awareness among adolescent males. *Family Planning Perspectives* 21(4):152-158, 1989.

88 Surveillance, Epidemiology, and End Results Program, 1987. National Cancer Institute, National Institutes of Health, Public Health Service, U.S. Department of Health and Human Services, Bethesda, MD.

89 Tabar, L.; Gad, A.; Holmberg L.H.; Ljungquist, V.; Eklund, G.; Fagorberg, C.J.G.; Baldetorp, L.; Grontoft, O.; Lundstrom, B.; Manson, J.C.; Day, N.E.; and Pehersson, F. Reduction in mortality from breast cancer after mass screening with mammography. *Lancet* 1:829-832, 1985.

90 Tanfer, K., and Horn, M.C. Contraceptive use, pregnancy, and fertility patterns among single American women in their 20s. *Family Planning Perspectives* 17(1):10-19, 1985.

91 U.S. Department of Agriculture and U.S. Department of Health and Human Services. *Dietary Guidelines for Americans.* Washington, DC: the Departments, 1990.

92 U.S. Preventive Services Task Force. *Guide to Clinical Preventive Services: An Assessment of the Effectiveness of 169 Interventions, Report of the U.S. Preventive Services Task Force.* Baltimore, MD: Williams and Wilkins, 1989.

93 Verbeek, A.L.M.; Hendricks, J.H.C.L.; Holland, R.; Mravunac, M.; Sturmans, F.; and Day, N.E. Reduction of breast cancer mortality through mass screening with modern mammography: First results of the Nijmegan Project, 1975-1981. *Lancet* 1:1222-1224, 1984.

94 Washington, A.E.; Arno, P.S.; and Brooks, M.A. The economic costs of pelvic inflammatory disease. *JAMA* 255:1735-1738, 1986.

95 Westat, Inc. *Study of the National Incidence of Child Abuse and Neglect.* Washington, DC: U.S. Department of Health and Human Services, 1988.

96 Woolhandler, S., and Himmelstein, D.U. Reverse targeting of preventive care due to lack of health insurance. *JAMA* 259:2872-2874, 1988.

6. Shared Responsibilities

The challenge set out through *Healthy People 2000* is one directed to people throughout the Nation. Each of us, whether acting as an individual, an employee or employer, a member of a family, community group, professional organization, or government agency, has both an opportunity and an obligation to contribute to the effort to improve the Nation's health profile. To arrive at the established goals and objectives, we must chart a common course that depends upon commitment and action from every level of our society. Then the challenge can be met.

Personal Responsibility

The individual is both the starting point and the ultimate target of the campaign towards *Healthy People 2000*. Through the many roles that each of us fulfills in our daily lives, we are afforded numerous opportunities for promoting health and preventing disease. With these opportunities, though, comes responsibility, and the first role we must all undertake is responsibility for our own personal health habits. Improving personal health behavior can count among the most potent means to prevent disease and promote health. Measurable decreases in risks to health can result from changes in diet, exercise, tobacco use, alcohol and other drug use, injury prevention behavior, and sexual habits, but each of us must choose to make these changes a personal priority.

Our worksites can provide a smoking cessation program and a fitness center, for example, but we have to enroll. Fast food chains can offer salads, but we have to choose them. Legislators can mandate food labeling, but we must care enough to read the labels. Our health care providers can provide the necessary screening tests and immunizations, but we must take the initiative to obtain them.

While the responsibility for change lies with each of us, it also lies with all of us, and individuals cannot be expected to act alone.

The Family

The family is the primary context in which health promoting activities occur and is therefore potentially the most immediate source of health-related support and education for the individual. It is in the context of the family that attitudes and behaviors regarding diet, physical activity, hygiene, smoking, and alcohol and other drug use are often learned and maintained. Therefore, the family offers the primary opportunity for change in these areas. Parents can teach children healthy habits and offer the supportive environment necessary to sustain them. In addition, parents can ensure that their children receive needed preventive services—immunizations, screening tests, as well as counseling and education about health risks and behaviors.

Although the family plays a key role in meeting the challenge of *Healthy People 2000*, the family also should not be expected to assume these responsibilities in isolation. Families need and deserve the support of their communities in achieving and maintaining standards of good health. When families experience stresses that can result in self-destruction through abuse, neglect, and addiction, the community's responsibility becomes increasingly urgent. Single-parent homes, children in poverty, and an aging society are all factors that threaten the family's viability. As the burdens of a family increase, its very spirit is threatened and the need for community support becomes still more crucial, not only to the well-being of its members but also to its survival.

Community

In today's society, a supportive community can make a vital difference in the well-being of its members. Accordingly, there is evidence that community-based health programs can play a strong role in improving the health status of their citizens. Multiple opportunities exist for community health promotion efforts on the part of government, voluntary and self-help groups, businesses, and schools. Such local community programs are often more efficient than centralized programs managed far from the point of delivery. Furthermore, indigenous programs maintain the sensitivity to family and neighborhood values that is vital to encourage change successfully towards healthier lifestyles within the community.

Local health officials can contribute to the challenge of *Healthy People 2000* by working to ensure that health department clinics provide appropriate preventive and health promotion services for the people they serve—in addition to their historic roles of providing and monitoring traditional community health services related to public sanitation, clean water, and water fluoridation. Local governments can form partnerships with grassroots organizations, such as neighborhood associations and tenant councils, in a cooperative effort to reach specific populations on topics of special local concern.

Voluntary organizations have long worked to improve health through research, public education, and other program activities. In fact, the spirit of volunteerism is one of our strongest national traditions. Groups that have not traditionally been involved in reducing health risks should now begin to define their role in community health education. For example, local organizations serving youth can collaborate on alcohol and other drug abuse-reduction programs or on discouraging the use of tobacco. Groups representing special populations—people with disabilities, racial and ethnic minorities, older people— can work together to achieve needed changes both within their memberships and in the community at large.

Business, community leaders, and labor can work together for mutual benefit to enhance the well-being of employees and the community. Management, unions, and employee groups can sponsor wellness and employee assistance programs; coverage for effective preventive services can be sought in contract negotiations; and employees can work to make community health promotion services available at the worksite for themselves, their dependents, and retirees. Many important disease prevention and health promotion activities, such as smoking cessation, diet modification, and physical conditioning, can be accomplished at the worksite in an effective and efficient manner. Company policies can help create a healthy work and living environment and contribute to the ecology of the communities in which they are based. From enforcing safety procedures, to mandating smoke-free workplaces, to ensuring that healthful food choices are available in employee cafeterias, employers have multiple opportunities to improve the health prospects of their employees. Companies also have a responsibility to contribute to the community leadership in maintaining a healthy environment through responsible waste disposal policies.

Schools have a special role in enhancing and maintaining the health of their community's children, since roughly one-quarter of a young person's time is spent in this environment. School health education can foster healthful behaviors and help prevent hazardous ones, particularly in the areas of physical fitness, smoking, and nutrition. Standard course curricula can be modified to include health promotion, as, for example, through the addition of environmental health components to science classes. Provision of healthy meals, safe work and play areas, and physical education courses that stress the acquisition of lifetime exercise habits can be instituted as well to foster the long-term health of our youth. In partnership with parents and other community groups, schools can help to create health promotion programs and enhance health education curricula. Schools can, in addition, open their facilities and health curricula to the adults of the community, thereby serving as an even greater local resource.

Churches and other religious institutions may also offer important resources for enhancing access to health promotion and disease prevention services, especially for populations that may otherwise be difficult to reach. Churches are often strong in the same communities where the health care system is weak and overburdened. In poor black communities, for example, the church has met not only the spiritual but also the educational, physical, and social needs of its members and their families and friends. Increasingly, religious institutions are sponsoring health fairs and establishing blood pressure education, screening, and control programs. They offer individual and family counseling and are often involved in adolescent pregnancy prevention efforts. These are important contributions.

Health Professionals

Responsibility also falls to physicians and other health care providers, who are for many Americans the primary sources of health information. Their professional training gives them the skill to translate science into practice. Practice can take the form of partnerships with nonprofessionals in the pursuit of individual, family, and community health care. The effectiveness and efficiency of preventive services—screening tests, immunizations, and counseling—will be enhanced by such partnerships.

Health education and counseling, in particular, provide opportunities for interdisciplinary consulting among educators, administrators, social workers, health and other professionals in order to integrate healthy practices into the daily lives of individuals, their families, and communities. Professional associations can facilitate dissemination of the health promotion and disease prevention knowledge base through their established information exchange and professional education networks. A special opportunity and responsibility exists for the teachers of health professionals to design curricula and allocate educational resources which will equip health-related professions with prevention expertise and with the skills to share their knowledge with the public.

America's physicians, dentists, nurses, pharmacists, medical technicians and other health professionals must be not only knowledgeable in the basic and clinical sciences; they also must be life-long learners, excellent communicators, good team players, managers of scarce resources, health care visionaries, and community leaders. The day of the solo practitioner, dealing with the patient in isolation from other professionals is past.

Media

The day of the print and electronic media is, however, very much here, and these media can contribute to the exchange of health information between health professionals and the public, as well as among health professionals themselves. The average American is exposed to many different kinds of health-related messages, some explicit in news, public affairs, and documentaries, and some buried in the plots and characters seen in entertainment programs through the mass media. In partnerships with the media, voluntary and professional organizations can expand the reach of their programs while performing an important service to the community.

Partnerships can also be created between community groups and the increasing number of cable television stations, radio stations, and regional magazines that are aimed at very specific audiences and therefore have a unique opportunity to tailor their messages directly to the target audience. New opportunities will also unfold through the evolving integration of telecommunications media—telephone, television, computer—to make customized health information more accessible than ever before.

Government

Policy decisions are made regularly that can assist health professionals and the public in reaching our national health goals. These decisions range from health care legislation to legislation that bears on the environment, business, farming, production, energy, housing, information dissemination, education, and the economy. The health interests of Americans are directly and indirectly shaped by such policy decisions. Local, State, and Federal governments can ensure that health promotion and disease prevention activities receive adequate attention and support. The accomplishment of this task can be effectively bridged through partnerships with each other and with the private sector.

With the increasing decentralization of government health services, the States have taken on new roles as conveners, fostering alliances and common interests among many potential participants in disease prevention and health promotion activities. These alliances can occur both horizontally, among statewide organizations, and vertically, among community, State, and national groups. Particularly important is their role in maintaining surveillance systems on the occurrence of disease, exposure to risks, and delivery of services. They are in this respect the keepers of the tools most important to charting our progress.

The Federal Government supports basic biomedical research on disease prevention and sponsors demonstration projects to help identify effective health promotion strategies. It provides financial support for many State and local government initiatives in health promotion and disease prevention, and directly serves some of the population groups most in need. On issues of particular prominence, it sponsors the development of national educational campaigns and the formation of coalitions for action. In order to address public health issues that are in flux with changing social, behavioral, and economic environments, sustained Federal leadership is necessary to improve the health of the American people.

Healthy People: The Vision

Clearly, to meet the challenge of the *Healthy People 2000* goals and objectives, we must work both individually and collectively. Alone, no one person, family, business, organization, or government has the resources to bring about the changes needed to implement this broad program, and yet the program cannot succeed unless each of us contributes individually. In essence, *Healthy People 2000* offers hope that through cooperative efforts all Americans can live longer, healthier lives.

There are existing examples of cooperative programs which, if replicated, could propel us toward our health goals for the year 2000. Promising efforts are emerging in programs that have taken deep roots in neighborhoods across America and focus upon the early developmental needs of children. In many areas, these programs are the chief, if not the only, agents of family and community. Through these efforts, parents can both receive support and become active participants and leaders within the community. Where such programs are successful, they demonstrate that by working together—by mobilizing families, neighborhoods, schools, businesses, churches, the media, and government—we can make great strides toward helping Americans become healthier, more productive, and more fulfilled.

Thus, the final message of this report is one of shared responsibility—among the many partners in prevention. It is what we do collectively and personally that will move us as individuals and as a Nation towards a healthier future.

Appendices

Contents

A. Summary List of Objectives

Duplicate objectives, which appear in two or more priority areas, are marked with an asterisk (*).

Except as otherwise noted, all rates in the following objectives are annual. Where the baseline rate is age adjusted, it is age adjusted to the 1940 U.S. population, and the target is age adjusted also.

1. Physical Activity And Fitness

Health Status Objectives

1.1* Reduce coronary heart disease deaths to no more than 100 per 100,000 people. (Age-adjusted baseline: 135 per 100,000 in 1987)

	Special Population Target	
Coronary Deaths (per 100,000)	*1987 Baseline*	*2000 Target*
1.1a Blacks	163	115

1.2* Reduce overweight to a prevalence of no more than 20 percent among people aged 20 and older and no more than 15 percent among adolescents aged 12 through 19. (Baseline: 26 percent for people aged 20 through 74 in 1976-80, 24 percent for men and 27 percent for women; 15 percent for adolescents aged 12 through 19 in 1976-80)

	Special Population Targets	
Overweight Prevalence	*1976-80 Baseline[†]*	*2000 Target*
1.2a Low-income women aged 20 and older	37%	25%
1.2b Black women aged 20 and older	44%	30%
1.2c Hispanic women aged 20 and older		25%
Mexican-American women	39%[‡]	
Cuban women	34%[‡]	
Puerto Rican women	37%[‡]	
1.2d American Indians/Alaska Natives	29-75%[§]	30%
1.2e People with disabilities	36%[+]	25%
1.2f Women with high blood pressure	50%	41%
1.2g Men with high blood pressure	39%	35%

[†]*Baseline for people aged 20-74* [‡]*1982-84 baseline for Hispanics aged 20-74*

[§]*1984-88 estimates for different tribes* [+]*1985 baseline for people aged 20-74 who report any limitation in activity due to chronic conditions*

Note: For people aged 20 and older, overweight is defined as body mass index (BMI) equal to or greater than 27.8 for men and 27.3 for women. For adolescents, overweight is defined as BMI equal to or greater than 23.0 for males aged 12 through 14, 24.3 for males aged 15 through 17, 25.8 for males aged 18 through 19, 23.4 for females aged 12 through 14, 24.8 for females aged 15 through 17, and 25.7 for females aged 18 through 19. The values for adolescents are the age- and gender-specific 85th percentile values of the 1976-80 National Health and Nutrition Examination Survey (NHANES II), corrected for sample variation. BMI is calculated by dividing weight in kilograms by the square of height in meters. The cut points used to define overweight approximate the 120 percent of desirable body weight definition used in the 1990 objectives.

Risk Reduction Objectives

1.3* Increase to at least 30 percent the proportion of people aged 6 and older who engage regularly, preferably daily, in light to moderate physical activity for at least 30 minutes per day. (Baseline: 22 percent of people aged 18 and older were active for at least 30 minutes 5 or more times per week and 12 percent were active 7 or more times per week in 1985)

Note: Light to moderate physical activity requires sustained, rhythmic muscular movements, is at least equivalent to sustained walking, and is performed at less than 60 percent of maximum heart rate for age. Maximum heart rate equals roughly 220 beats per minute minus age. Examples may include walking, swimming, cycling, dancing, gardening and yardwork, various domestic and occupational activities, and games and other childhood pursuits.

1.4   Increase to at least 20 percent the proportion of people aged 18 and older and to at least 75 percent the proportion of children and adolescents aged 6 through 17 who engage in vigorous physical activity that promotes the development and maintenance of cardiorespiratory fitness 3 or more days per week for 20 or more minutes per occasion. (Baseline: 12 percent for people aged 18 and older in 1985; 66 percent for youth aged 10 through 17 in 1984)

	Special Population Target	
Vigorous Physical Activity	*1985 Baseline*	*2000 Target*
1.4a Lower-income people aged 18 and older (annual family income <$20,000)	7%	12%

Note: Vigorous physical activities are rhythmic, repetitive physical activities that use large muscle groups at 60 percent or more of maximum heart rate for age. An exercise heart rate of 60 percent of maximum heart rate for age is about 50 percent of maximal cardiorespiratory capacity and is sufficient for cardiorespiratory conditioning. Maximum heart rate equals roughly 220 beats per minute minus age.

1.5   Reduce to no more than 15 percent the proportion of people aged 6 and older who engage in no leisure-time physical activity. (Baseline: 24 percent for people aged 18 and older in 1985)

	Special Population Targets	
No Leisure-Time Physical Activity	*1985 Baseline*	*2000 Target*
1.5a People aged 65 and older	43%	22%
1.5b People with disabilities	35%[†]	20%
1.5c Lower-income people (annual family income <$20,000)	32%[†]	17%

[†]*Baseline for people aged 18 and older*

Note: For this objective, people with disabilities are people who report any limitation in activity due to chronic conditions.

1.6   Increase to at least 40 percent the proportion of people aged 6 and older who regularly perform physical activities that enhance and maintain muscular strength, muscular endurance, and flexibility. (Baseline data available in 1991)

1.7*   Increase to at least 50 percent the proportion of overweight people aged 12 and older who have adopted sound dietary practices combined with regular physical activity to attain an appropriate body weight. (Baseline: 30 percent of overweight women and 25 percent of overweight men for people aged 18 and older in 1985)

Services and Protection Objectives

1.8   Increase to at least 50 percent the proportion of children and adolescents in 1st through 12th grade who participate in daily school physical education. (Baseline: 36 percent in 1984-86)

1.9   Increase to at least 50 percent the proportion of school physical education class time that students spend being physically active, preferably engaged in lifetime physical activities. (Baseline: Students spent an estimated 27 percent of class time being physically active in 1983)

Note: Lifetime activities are activities that may be readily carried into adulthood because they generally need only one or two people. Examples include swimming, bicycling, jogging, and racquet sports. Also counted as lifetime activities are vigorous social activities such as dancing. Competitive group sports and activities typically played only by young children such as group games are excluded.

1.10   Increase the proportion of worksites offering employer-sponsored physical activity and fitness programs as follows:

Worksite Size	*1985 Baseline*	*2000 Target*
50-99 employees	14%	20%
100-249 employees	23%	35%
250-749 employees	32%	50%
≥750 employees	54%	80%

1.11   Increase community availability and accessibility of physical activity and fitness facilities as follows:

Facility	*1986 Baseline*	*2000 Target*
Hiking, biking, and fitness trail miles	1 per 71,000 people	1 per 10,000 people
Public swimming pools	1 per 53,000 people	1 per 25,000 people
Acres of park and recreation open space	1.8 per 1,000 people (553 people per managed acre)	4 per 1,000 people (250 people per managed acre)

1.12   Increase to at least 50 percent the proportion of primary care providers who routinely assess and counsel their patients regarding the frequency, duration, type, and intensity of each patient's physical activity practices. (Baseline: Physicians provided exercise counseling for about 30 percent of sedentary patients in 1988)

2. Nutrition

Health Status Objectives

2.1* Reduce coronary heart disease deaths to no more than 100 per 100,000 people. (Age-adjusted baseline: 135 per 100,000 in 1987)

Special Population Target

Coronary Deaths (per 100,000)	*1987 Baseline*	*2000 Target*
2.1a Blacks	163	115

2.2* Reverse the rise in cancer deaths to achieve a rate of no more than 130 per 100,000 people. (Age-adjusted baseline: 133 per 100,000 in 1987)

Note: In its publications, the National Cancer Institute age adjusts cancer death rates to the 1970 U.S. population. Using the 1970 standard, the equivalent baseline and target values for this objective would be 171 and 175 per 100,000, respectively.

2.3* Reduce overweight to a prevalence of no more than 20 percent among people aged 20 and older and no more than 15 percent among adolescents aged 12 through 19. (Baseline: 26 percent for people aged 20 through 74 in 1976-80, 24 percent for men and 27 percent for women; 15 percent for adolescents aged 12 through 19 in 1976-80)

Special Population Targets

Overweight Prevalence	*1976-80 Baseline[†]*	*2000 Target*
2.3a Low-income women aged 20 and older	37%	25%
2.3b Black women aged 20 and older	44%	30%
2.3c Hispanic women aged 20 and older		25%
Mexican-American women	39%[‡]	
Cuban women	34%[‡]	
Puerto Rican women	37%[‡]	
2.3d American Indians/Alaska Natives	29-75%[§]	30%
2.3e People with disabilities	36%[+]	25%
2.3f Women with high blood pressure	50%	41%
2.3g Men with high blood pressure	39%	35%

[†]*Baseline for people aged 20-74* [‡]*1982-84 baseline for Hispanics aged 20-74*
[§]*1984-88 estimates for different tribes* [+]*1985 baseline for people aged 20-74 who report any limitation in activity due to chronic conditions*

Note: For people aged 20 and older, overweight is defined as body mass index (BMI) equal to or greater than 27.8 for men and 27.3 for women. For adolescents, overweight is defined as BMI equal to or greater than 23.0 for males aged 12 through 14, 24.3 for males aged 15 through 17, 25.8 for males aged 18 through 19, 23.4 for females aged 12 through 14, 24.8 for females aged 15 through 17, and 25.7 for females aged 18 through 19. The values for adolescents are the age- and gender-specific 85th percentile values of the 1976-80 National Health and Nutrition Examination Survey (NHANES II), corrected for sample variation. BMI is calculated by dividing weight in kilograms by the square of height in meters. The cut points used to define overweight approximate the 120 percent of desirable body weight definition used in the 1990 objectives.

2.4 Reduce growth retardation among low-income children aged 5 and younger to less than 10 percent. (Baseline: Up to 16 percent among low-income children in 1988, depending on age and race/ethnicity)

Special Population Targets

Prevalence of Short Stature	*1988 Baseline*	*2000 Target*
2.4a Low-income black children <age 1	15%	10%
2.4b Low-income Hispanic children <age 1	13%	10%
2.4c Low-income Hispanic children aged 1	16%	10%
2.4d Low-income Asian/Pacific Islander children aged 1	14%	10%
2.4e Low-income Asian/Pacific Islander children aged 2-4	16%	10%

Note: Growth retardation is defined as height-for-age below the fifth percentile of children in the National Center for Health Statistics' reference population.

Risk Reduction Objectives

2.5* Reduce dietary fat intake to an average of 30 percent of calories or less and average saturated fat intake to less than 10 percent of calories among people aged 2 and older. (Baseline: 36 percent of calories from total fat and 13 percent from saturated fat for people aged 20 through 74 in 1976-80; 36 percent and 13 percent for women aged 19 through 50 in 1985)

2.6* Increase complex carbohydrate and fiber-containing foods in the diets of adults to 5 or more daily servings for vegetables (including legumes) and fruits, and to 6 or more daily servings for grain products. (Baseline: 2½ servings of vegetables and fruits and 3 servings of grain products for women aged 19 through 50 in 1985)

2.7* Increase to at least 50 percent the proportion of overweight people aged 12 and older who have adopted sound dietary practices combined with regular physical activity to attain an appropriate body weight. (Baseline: 30 percent of overweight women and 25 percent of overweight men for people aged 18 and older in 1985)

2.8   Increase calcium intake so at least 50 percent of youth aged 12 through 24 and 50 percent of pregnant and lactating women consume 3 or more servings daily of foods rich in calcium, and at least 50 percent of people aged 25 and older consume 2 or more servings daily. (Baseline: 7 percent of women and 14 percent of men aged 19 though 24 and 24 percent of pregnant and lactating women consumed 3 or more servings, and 15 percent of women and 23 percent of men aged 25 through 50 consumed 2 or more servings in 1985-86)

Note: The number of servings of foods rich in calcium is based on milk and milk products. A serving is considered to be 1 cup of skim milk or its equivalent in calcium (302 mg). The number of servings in this objective will generally provide approximately three-fourths of the 1989 Recommended Dietary Allowance (RDA) of calcium. The RDA is 1200 mg for people aged 12 through 24, 800 mg for people aged 25 and older, and 1200 mg for pregnant and lactating women.

2.9   Decrease salt and sodium intake so at least 65 percent of home meal preparers prepare foods without adding salt, at least 80 percent of people avoid using salt at the table, and at least 40 percent of adults regularly purchase foods modified or lower in sodium. (Baseline: 54 percent of women aged 19 through 50 who served as the main meal preparer did not use salt in food preparation, and 68 percent of women aged 19 through 50 did not use salt at the table in 1985; 20 percent of all people aged 18 and older regularly purchased foods with reduced salt and sodium content in 1988)

2.10   Reduce iron deficiency to less than 3 percent among children aged 1 through 4 and among women of childbearing age. (Baseline: 9 percent for children aged 1 through 2, 4 percent for children aged 3 through 4, and 5 percent for women aged 20 through 44 in 1976-80)

Special Population Targets

Iron Deficiency Prevalence	1976-80 Baseline	2000 Target
2.10a Low-income children aged 1-2	21%	10%
2.10b Low-income children aged 3-4	10%	5%
2.10c Low-income women of childbearing age	8%[†]	4%

Anemia Prevalence	1983-85 Baseline	2000 Target
2.10d Alaska Native children aged 1-5	22-28%	10%
2.10e Black, low-income pregnant women (third trimester)	41%[‡]	20%

[†]*Baseline for women aged 20-44*   [‡]*1988 baseline for women aged 15-44*

Note: Iron deficiency is defined as having abnormal results for 2 or more of the following tests: mean corpuscular volume, erythrocyte protoporphyrin, and transferrin saturation. Anemia is used as an index of iron deficiency. Anemia among Alaska Native children was defined as hemoglobin <11 gm/dL or hematocrit <34 percent. For pregnant women in the third trimester, anemia was defined according to CDC criteria. The above prevalences of iron deficiency and anemia may be due to inadequate dietary iron intakes or to inflammatory conditions and infections. For anemia, genetics may also be a factor.

2.11* Increase to at least 75 percent the proportion of mothers who breastfeed their babies in the early postpartum period and to at least 50 percent the proportion who continue breastfeeding until their babies are 5 to 6 months old. (Baseline: 54 percent at discharge from birth site and 21 percent at 5 to 6 months in 1988)

Special Population Targets

Mothers Breastfeeding Their Babies:	1988 Baseline	2000 Target
During Early Postpartum Period—		
2.11a Low-income mothers	32%	75%
2.11b Black mothers	25%	75%
2.11c Hispanic mothers	51%	75%
2.11d American Indian/Alaska Native mothers	47%	75%
At Age 5-6 Months—		
2.11a Low-income mothers	9%	50%
2.11b Black mothers	8%	50%
2.11c Hispanic mothers	16%	50%
2.11d American Indian/Alaska Native mothers	28%	50%

2.12* Increase to at least 75 percent the proportion of parents and caregivers who use feeding practices that prevent baby bottle tooth decay. (Baseline data available in 1991)

Special Population Targets

Appropriate Feeding Practices	Baseline	2000 Target
2.12a Parents and caregivers with less than high school education	—	65%
2.12b American Indian/Alaska Native parents and caregivers	—	65%

2.13   Increase to at least 85 percent the proportion of people aged 18 and older who use food labels to make nutritious food selections. (Baseline: 74 percent used labels to make food selections in 1988)

Services and Protection Objectives

2.14   Achieve useful and informative nutrition labeling for virtually all processed foods and at least 40 percent of fresh meats, poultry, fish, fruits, vegetables, baked goods, and ready-to-eat carry-away foods. (Baseline: 60 percent of sales of processed foods regulated by FDA had nutrition labeling in 1988; baseline data on fresh and carry-away foods unavailable)

2.15 Increase to at least 5,000 brand items the availability of processed food products that are reduced in fat and saturate fat. (Baseline: 2,500 items reduced in fat in 1986)

Note: A brand item is defined as a particular flavor and/or size of a specific brand and is typically the consumer unit of purchase.

2.16 Increase to at least 90 percent the proportion of restaurants and institutional food service operations that offer identifiable low-fat, low-calorie food choices, consistent with the *Dietary Guidelines for Americans.* (Baseline: About 70 percent of fast food and family restaurant chains with 350 or more units had at least one low-fat, low-calorie item on their menu in 1989)

2.17 Increase to at least 90 percent the proportion of school lunch and breakfast services and child care food services with menus that are consistent with the nutrition principles in the *Dietary Guidelines for Americans.* (Baseline data available in 1993)

2.18 Increase to at least 80 percent the receipt of home food services by people aged 65 and older who have difficulty in preparing their own meals or are otherwise in need of home-delivered meals. (Baseline data available in 1991)

2.19 Increase to at least 75 percent the proportion of the Nation's schools that provide nutrition education from preschool through 12th grade, preferably as part of quality school health education. (Baseline data available in 1991)

2.20 Increase to at least 50 percent the proportion of worksites with 50 or more employees that offer nutrition education and/or weight management programs for employees. (Baseline: 17 percent offered nutrition education activities and 15 percent offered weight control activities in 1985)

2.21 Increase to at least 75 percent the proportion of primary care providers who provide nutrition assessment and counseling and/or referral to qualified nutritionists or dietitians. (Baseline: Physicians provided diet counseling for an estimated 40 to 50 percent of patients in 1988)

3. Tobacco

Health Status Objectives

3.1* Reduce coronary heart disease deaths to no more than 100 per 100,000 people. (Age-adjusted baseline: 135 per 100,000 in 1987)

Special Population Target

Coronary Deaths (per 100,000)		*1987 Baseline*	*2000 Target*
3.1a	Blacks	163	115

3.2* Slow the rise in lung cancer deaths to achieve a rate of no more than 42 per 100,000 people. (Age-adjusted baseline: 37.9 per 100,000 in 1987)

Note: In its publications, the National Cancer Institute age adjusts cancer death rates to the 1970 U.S. population. Using the 1970 standard, the equivalent baseline and target values for this objective would be 47.9 and 53 per 100,000, respectively.

3.3 Slow the rise in deaths from chronic obstructive pulmonary disease to achieve a rate of no more than 25 per 100,000 people. (Age-adjusted baseline: 18.7 per 100,000 in 1987)

Note: Deaths from chronic obstructive pulmonary disease include deaths due to chronic bronchitis, emphysema, asthma, and other chronic obstructive pulmonary diseases and allied conditions.

Risk Reduction Objectives

3.4* Reduce cigarette smoking to a prevalence of no more than 15 percent among people aged 20 and older. (Baseline: 29 percent in 1987, 32 percent for men and 27 percent for women)

Special Population Targets

	Cigarette Smoking Prevalence	*1987 Baseline*	*2000 Target*
3.4a	People with a high school education or less aged 20 and older	34%	20%
3.4b	Blue-collar workers aged 20 and older	36%	20%
3.4c	Military personnel	42%[†]	20%
3.4d	Blacks aged 20 and older	34%	18%
3.4e	Hispanics aged 20 and older	33%[‡]	18%
3.4f	American Indians/Alaska Natives	42-70%[§]	20%
3.4g	Southeast Asian men	55%[+]	20%
3.4h	Women of reproductive age	29%[††]	12%
3.4i	Pregnant women	25%[‡‡]	10%
3.4j	Women who use oral contraceptives	36%[§§]	10%

[†]*1988 baseline* [‡]*1982-84 baseline for Hispanics aged 20-74* [§]*1979-87 estimates for different tribes*
[+]*1984-88 baseline* [††]*Baseline for women aged 18-44* [‡‡]*1985 baseline* [§§]*1983 baseline*

Note: A cigarette smoker is a person who has smoked at least 100 cigarettes and currently smokes cigarettes.

3.5 Reduce the initiation of cigarette smoking by children and youth so that no more than 15 percent have become regular cigarette smokers by age 20. (Baseline: 30 percent of youth had become regular cigarette smokers by ages 20 through 24 in 1987)

Special Population Target

Initiation of Smoking	1987 Baseline	2000 Target
3.5a Lower socioeconomic status youth[†]	40%	18%

[†]*As measured by people aged 20-24 with a high school education or less*

3.6 Increase to at least 50 percent the proportion of cigarette smokers aged 18 and older who stopped smoking cigarettes for at least one day during the preceding year. (Baseline: In 1986, 34 percent of people who smoked in the preceding year stopped for at least one day during that year)

3.7 Increase smoking cessation during pregnancy so that at least 60 percent of women who are cigarette smokers at the time they become pregnant quit smoking early in pregnancy and maintain abstinence for the remainder of their pregnancy. (Baseline: 39 percent of white women aged 20 through 44 quit at any time during pregnancy in 1985)

Special Population Target

Cessation and Abstinence During Pregnancy	1985 Baseline	2000 Target
3.7a Women with less than a high school education	28%[†]	45%

[†]*Baseline for white women aged 20-44*

3.8 Reduce to no more than 20 percent the proportion of children aged 6 and younger who are regularly exposed to tobacco smoke at home. (Baseline: More than 39 percent in 1986, as 39 percent of households with one or more children aged 6 or younger had a cigarette smoker in the household)

Note: Regular exposure to tobacco smoke at home is defined as the occurrence of tobacco smoking anywhere in the home on more than 3 days each week.

3.9 Reduce smokeless tobacco use by males aged 12 through 24 to a prevalence of no more than 4 percent. (Baseline: 6.6 percent among males aged 12 through 17 in 1988; 8.9 percent among males aged 18 through 24 in 1987)

Special Population Target

Smokeless Tobacco Use	1986-87 Baseline	2000 Target
3.9a American Indian/Alaska Native youth	18-64%	10%

Note: For males aged 12 through 17, a smokeless tobacco user is someone who has used snuff or chewing tobacco in the preceding month. For males aged 18 through 24, a smokeless tobacco user is someone who has used either snuff or chewing tobacco at least 20 times and who currently uses snuff or chewing tobacco.

Services and Protection Objectives

3.10 Establish tobacco-free environments and include tobacco use prevention in the curricula of all elementary, middle, and secondary schools, preferably as part of quality school health education. (Baseline: 17 percent of school districts totally banned smoking on school premises or at school functions in 1988; antismoking education was provided by 78 percent of school districts at the high school level, 81 percent at the middle school level, and 75 percent at the elementary school level in 1988)

3.11 Increase to at least 75 percent the proportion of worksites with a formal smoking policy that prohibits or severely restricts smoking at the workplace. (Baseline: 27 percent of worksites with 50 or more employees in 1985; 54 percent of medium and large companies in 1987)

3.12 Enact in 50 States comprehensive laws on clean indoor air that prohibit or strictly limit smoking in the workplace and enclosed public places (including health care facilities, schools, and public transportation). (Baseline: 42 States and the District of Columbia had laws restricting smoking in public places; 31 States restricted smoking in public workplaces; but only 13 States had comprehensive laws regulating smoking in private as well as public worksites and at least 4 public places, including restaurants, as of 1988)

3.13 Enact and enforce in 50 States laws prohibiting the sale and distribution of tobacco products to youth younger than age 19. (Baseline: 44 States and the District of Columbia had, but rarely enforced, laws regulating the sale and/or distribution of cigarettes or tobacco products to minors in 1990; only 3 set the age of majority at 19 and only 6 prohibited cigarette vending machines accessible to minors)

Note: Model legislation proposed by DHHS recommends licensure of tobacco vendors, civil money penalties and license suspension or revocation for violations, and a ban on cigarette vending machines.

3.14 Increase to 50 the number of States with plans to reduce tobacco use, especially among youth. (Baseline: 12 States in 1989)

3.15 Eliminate or severely restrict all forms of tobacco product advertising and promotion to which youth younger than age 18 are likely to be exposed. (Baseline: Radio and television advertising of tobacco products were prohibited, but other restrictions on advertising and promotion to which youth may be exposed were minimal in 1990)

3.16 Increase to at least 75 percent the proportion of primary care and oral health care providers who routinely advise cessation and provide assistance and followup for all of their tobacco-using patients. (Baseline: About 52 percent of internists reported counseling more than 75 percent of their smoking patients about smoking cessation in 1986; about 35 percent of dentists reported counseling at least 75 percent of their smoking patients about smoking in 1986)

4. Alcohol and Other Drugs

Health Status Objectives

4.1 Reduce deaths caused by alcohol-related motor vehicle crashes to no more than 8.5 per 100,000 people. (Age-adjusted baseline: 9.8 per 100,000 in 1987)

Special Population Targets

Alcohol-Related Motor Vehicle Crash Deaths (per 100,000)	1987 Baseline	2000 Target
4.1a American Indian/Alaska Native men	52.2	44.8
4.1b People aged 15-24	21.5	18

4.2 Reduce cirrhosis deaths to no more than 6 per 100,000 people. (Age-adjusted baseline: 9.1 per 100,000 in 1987)

Special Population Targets

Cirrhosis Deaths (per 100,000)	1987 Baseline	2000 Target
4.2a Black men	22	12
4.2b American Indians/Alaska Natives	25.9	13

4.3 Reduce drug-related deaths to no more than 3 per 100,000 people. (Age-adjusted baseline: 3.8 per 100,000 in 1987)

4.4 Reduce drug abuse-related hospital emergency department visits by at least 20 percent. (Baseline data available in 1991)

Risk Reduction Objectives

4.5 Increase by at least 1 year the average age of first use of cigarettes, alcohol, and marijuana by adolescents aged 12 through 17. (Baseline: Age 11.6 for cigarettes, age 13.1 for alcohol, and age 13.4 for marijuana in 1988)

4.6 Reduce the proportion of young people who have used alcohol, marijuana, and cocaine in the past month, as follows:

Substance/Age	1988 Baseline	2000 Target
Alcohol/aged 12-17	25.2%	12.6%
Alcohol/aged 18-20	57.9%	29%
Marijuana/aged 12-17	6.4%	3.2%
Marijuana/aged 18-25	15.5%	7.8%
Cocaine/aged 12-17	1.1%	0.6%
Cocaine/aged 18-25	4.5%	2.3%

Note: The targets of this objective are consistent with the goals established by the Office of National Drug Control Policy, Executive Office of the President.

4.7 Reduce the proportion of high school seniors and college students engaging in recent occasions of heavy drinking of alcoholic beverages to no more than 28 percent of high school seniors and 32 percent of college students. (Baseline: 33 percent of high school seniors and 41.7 percent of college students in 1989)

Note: Recent heavy drinking is defined as having 5 or more drinks on one occasion in the previous 2-week period as monitored by self-reports.

4.8 Reduce alcohol consumption by people aged 14 and older to an annual average of no more than 2 gallons of ethanol per person. (Baseline: 2.54 gallons of ethanol in 1987)

4.9 Increase the proportion of high school seniors who perceive social disapproval associated with the heavy use of alcohol, occasional use of marijuana, and experimentation with cocaine, as follows:

Behavior	1989 Baseline	2000 Target
Heavy use of alcohol	56.4%	70%
Occasional use of marijuana	71.1%	85%
Trying cocaine once or twice	88.9%	95%

Note: Heavy drinking is defined as having 5 or more drinks once or twice each weekend.

4.10 Increase the proportion of high school seniors who associate risk of physical or psychological harm with the heavy use of alcohol, regular use of marijuana, and experimentation with cocaine, as follows:

Behavior	1989 Baseline	2000 Target
Heavy use of alcohol	44%	70%
Regular use of marijuana	77.5%	90%
Trying cocaine once or twice	54.9%	80%

Note: Heavy drinking is defined as having 5 or more drinks once or twice each weekend.

4.11 Reduce to no more than 3 percent the proportion of male high school seniors who use anabolic steroids. (Baseline: 4.7 percent in 1989)

Services and Protection Objectives

4.12 Establish and monitor in 50 States comprehensive plans to ensure access to alcohol and drug treatment programs for traditionally underserved people. (Baseline data available in 1991)

4.13 Provide to children in all school districts and private schools primary and secondary school educational programs on alcohol and other drugs, preferably as part of quality school health education. (Baseline: 63 percent provided some instruction, 39 percent provided counseling, and 23 percent referred students for clinical assessments in 1987)

4.14 Extend adoption of alcohol and drug policies for the work environment to at least 60 percent of worksites with 50 or more employees. (Baseline data available in 1991)

4.15 Extend to 50 States administrative driver's license suspension/revocation laws or programs of equal effectiveness for people determined to have been driving under the influence of intoxicants. (Baseline: 28 States and the District of Columbia in 1990)

4.16 Increase to 50 the number of States that have enacted and enforce policies, beyond those in existence in 1989, to reduce access to alcoholic beverages by minors.

Note: Policies to reduce access to alcoholic beverages by minors may include those that address restriction of the sale of alcoholic beverages at recreational and entertainment events at which youth make up a majority of participants/consumers, product pricing, penalties and license-revocation for sale of alcoholic beverages to minors, and other approaches designed to discourage and restrict purchase of alcoholic beverages by minors.

4.17 Increase to at least 20 the number of States that have enacted statutes to restrict promotion of alcoholic beverages that is focused principally on young audiences. (Baseline data available in 1992)

4.18 Extend to 50 States legal blood alcohol concentration tolerance levels of .04 percent for motor vehicle drivers aged 21 and older and .00 percent for those younger than age 21. (Baseline: 0 States in 1990)

4.19 Increase to at least 75 percent the proportion of primary care providers who screen for alcohol and other drug use problems and provide counseling and referral as needed. (Baseline data available in 1992)

5. Family Planning

Health Status Objectives

5.1 Reduce pregnancies among girls aged 17 and younger to no more than 50 per 1,000 adolescents. (Baseline: 71.1 pregnancies per 1,000 girls aged 15 through 17 in 1985)

	Special Population Targets	
Pregnancies (per 1,000)	*1985 Baseline*	*2000 Target*
5.1a Black adolescent girls aged 15-19	186[†]	120
5.1b Hispanic adolescent girls aged 15-19	158	105
[†]*Non-white adolescents*		

Note: For black and Hispanic adolescent girls, baseline data are unavailable for those aged 15 through 17. The targets for these two populations are based on data for women aged 15 through 19. If more complete data become available, a 35-percent reduction from baseline figures should be used as the target.

5.2 Reduce to no more than 30 percent the proportion of all pregnancies that are unintended. (Baseline: 56 percent of pregnancies in the previous 5 years were unintended, either unwanted or earlier than desired, in 1988)

	Special Population Target	
Unintended Pregnancies	*1988 Baseline*	*2000 Target*
5.2a Black women	78%	40%

5.3 Reduce the prevalence of infertility to no more than 6.5 percent. (Baseline: 7.9 percent of married couples with wives aged 15 through 44 in 1988)

	Special Population Targets	
Prevalence of Infertility	*1988 Baseline*	*2000 Target*
5.3a Black couples	12.1%	9%
5.3b Hispanic couples	12.4%	9%

Note: Infertility is the failure of couples to conceive after 12 months of intercourse without contraception.

Risk Reduction Objectives

5.4* Reduce the proportion of adolescents who have engaged in sexual intercourse to no more than 15 percent by age 15 and no more than 40 percent by age 17. (Baseline: 27 percent of girls and 33 percent of boys by age 15; 50 percent of girls and 66 percent of boys by age 17; reported in 1988)

5.5 Increase to at least 40 percent the proportion of ever sexually active adolescents aged 17 and younger who have abstained from sexual activity for the previous 3 months. (Baseline: 26 percent of sexually active girls aged 15 through 17 in 1988)

5.6 Increase to at least 90 percent the proportion of sexually active, unmarried people aged 19 and younger who use contraception, especially combined method contraception that both effectively prevents pregnancy and provides barrier protection against disease. (Baseline: 78 percent at most recent intercourse and 63 percent at first intercourse; 2 percent used oral contraceptives and the condom at most recent intercourse; among young women aged 15 through 19 reporting in 1988)

Note: Strategies to achieve this objective must be undertaken sensitively to avoid indirectly encouraging or condoning sexual activity among teens who are not yet sexually active.

5.7 Increase the effectiveness with which family planning methods are used, as measured by a decrease to no more than 5 percent in the proportion of couples experiencing pregnancy despite use of a contraceptive method. (Baseline: Approximately 10 percent of women using reversible contraceptive methods experienced an unintended pregnancy in 1982)

Services and Protection Objectives

5.8 Increase to at least 85 percent the proportion of people aged 10 through 18 who have discussed human sexuality, including values surrounding sexuality, with their parents and/or have received information through another parentally endorsed source, such as youth, school, or religious programs. (Baseline: 66 percent of people aged 13 through 18 have discussed sexuality with their parents; reported in 1986)

Note: This objective, which supports family communication on a range of vital personal health issues, will be tracked using the National Health Interview Survey, a continuing, voluntary, national sample survey of adults who report on household characteristics including such items as illnesses, injuries, use of health services, and demographic characteristics.

5.9 Increase to at least 90 percent the proportion of pregnancy counselors who offer positive, accurate information about adoption to their unmarried patients with unintended pregnancies. (Baseline: 60 percent of pregnancy counselors in 1984)

Note: Pregnancy counselors are any providers of health or social services who discuss the management or outcome of pregnancy with a woman after she has received a diagnosis of pregnancy.

5.10* Increase to at least 60 percent the proportion of primary care providers who provide age-appropriate preconception care and counseling. (Baseline data available in 1992)

5.11* Increase to at least 50 percent the proportion of family planning clinics, maternal and child health clinics, sexually transmitted disease clinics, tuberculosis clinics, drug treatment centers, and primary care clinics that screen, diagnose, treat, counsel, and provide (or refer for) partner notification services for HIV infection and bacterial sexually transmitted diseases (gonorrhea, syphilis, and chlamydia). (Baseline: 40 percent of family planning clinics for bacterial sexually transmitted diseases in 1989)

6. Mental Health and Mental Disorders

Health Status Objectives

6.1* Reduce suicides to no more than 10.5 per 100,000 people. (Age-adjusted baseline: 11.7 per 100,000 in 1987)

Special Population Targets

Suicides (per 100,000)	1987 Baseline	2000 Target
6.1a Youth aged 15-19	10.3	8.2
6.1b Men aged 20-34	25.2	21.4
6.1c White men aged 65 and older	46.1	39.2
6.1d American Indian/Alaska Native men in Reservation States	15	12.8

6.2* Reduce by 15 percent the incidence of injurious suicide attempts among adolescents aged 14 through 17. (Baseline data available in 1991)

6.3 Reduce to less than ? 0 percent the prevalence of mental disorders among children and adolescents. (Baseline: An estimated 12 percent among youth younger than age 18 in 1989)

6.4 Reduce the prevalence of mental disorders (exclusive of substance abuse) among adults living in the community to less than 10.7 percent. (Baseline: One-month point prevalence of 12.6 percent in 1984)

6.5 Reduce to less than 35 percent the proportion of people aged 18 and older who experienced adverse health effects from stress within the past year. (Baseline: 42.6 percent in 1985)

Special Population Target

	1985 Baseline	2000 Target
6.5a People with disabilities	53.5%	40%

Note: For this objective, people with disabilities are people who report any limitation in activity due to chronic conditions.

Risk Reduction Objectives

6.6 Increase to at least 30 percent the proportion of people aged 18 and older with severe, persistent mental disorders who use community support programs. (Baseline: 15 percent in 1986)

6.7 Increase to at least 45 percent the proportion of people with major depressive disorders who obtain treatment. (Baseline: 31 percent in 1982)

6.8   Increase to at least 20 percent the proportion of people aged 18 and older who seek help in coping with personal and emotional problems. (Baseline: 11.1 percent in 1985)

Special Population Target

	1985 Baseline	2000 Target
6.8a People with disabilities	14.7%	30%

6.9   Decrease to no more than 5 percent the proportion of people aged 18 and older who report experiencing significant levels of stress who do not take steps to reduce or control their stress. (Baseline: 21 percent in 1985)

Services and Protection Objectives

6.10*   Increase to 50 the number of States with officially established protocols that engage mental health, alcohol and drug, and public health authorities with corrections authorities to facilitate identification and appropriate intervention to prevent suicide by jail inmates. (Baseline data available in 1992)

6.11   Increase to at least 40 percent the proportion of worksites employing 50 or more people that provide programs to reduce employee stress. (Baseline: 26.6 percent in 1985)

6.12   Establish mutual help clearinghouses in at least 25 States. (Baseline: 9 States in 1989)

6.13   Increase to at least 50 percent the proportion of primary care providers who routinely review with patients their patients' cognitive, emotional, and behavioral functioning and the resources available to deal with any problems that are identified. (Baseline data available in 1992)

6.14   Increase to at least 75 percent the proportion of providers of primary care for children who include assessment of cognitive, emotional, and parent-child functioning, with appropriate counseling, referral, and followup, in their clinical practices. (Baseline data available in 1992)

7. Violent and Abusive Behavior

Health Status Objectives

7.1   Reduce homicides to no more than 7.2 per 100,000 people. (Age-adjusted baseline: 8.5 per 100,000 in 1987)

Special Population Targets

Homicide Rate (per 100,000)	1987 Baseline	2000 Target
7.1a Children aged 3 and younger	3.9	3.1
7.1b Spouses aged 15-34	1.7	1.4
7.1c Black men aged 15-34	90.5	72.4
7.1d Hispanic men aged 15-34	53.1	42.5
7.1e Black women aged 15-34	20.0	16.0
7.1f American Indians/Alaska Natives in Reservation States	14.1	11.3

7.2*   Reduce suicides to no more than 10.5 per 100,000 people. (Age-adjusted baseline: 11.7 per 100,000 in 1987)

Special Population Targets

Suicides (per 100,000)	1987 Baseline	2000 Target
7.2a Youth aged 15-19	10.3	8.2
7.2b Men aged 20-34	25.2	21.4
7.2c White men aged 65 and older	46.1	39.2
7.2d American Indian/Alaska Native men in Reservation States	15	12.8

7.3   Reduce weapon-related violent deaths to no more than 12.6 per 100,000 people from major causes. (Age-adjusted baseline: 12.9 per 100,000 by firearms, 1.9 per 100,000 by knives, in 1987)

7.4   Reverse to less than 25.2 per 1,000 children the rising incidence of maltreatment of children younger than age 18. (Baseline: 25.2 per 1,000 in 1986)

Type-Specific Targets

Incidence of Types of Maltreatment (per 1,000)	1986 Baseline	2000 Target
7.4a Physical abuse	5.7	<5.7
7.4b Sexual abuse	2.5	<2.5
7.4c Emotional abuse	3.4	<3.4
7.4d Neglect	15.9	<15.9

7.5   Reduce physical abuse directed at women by male partners to no more than 27 per 1,000 couples. (Baseline: 30 per 1,000 in 1985)

7.6   Reduce assault injuries among people aged 12 and older to no more than 10 per 1,000 people. (Baseline: 11.1 per 1,000 in 1986)

7.7   Reduce rape and attempted rape of women aged 12 and older to no more than 108 per 100,000 women. (Baseline: 120 per 100,000 in 1986)

Special Population Target

Incidence of Rape and Attempted Rape (per 100,000)	1986 Baseline	2000 Target
7.7a Women aged 12-34	250	225

7.8*   Reduce by 15 percent the incidence of injurious suicide attempts among adolescents aged 14 through 17. (Baseline data available in 1991)

Risk Reduction Objectives

7.9   Reduce by 20 percent the incidence of physical fighting among adolescents aged 14 through 17. (Baseline data available in 1991)

7.10   Reduce by 20 percent the incidence of weapon-carrying by adolescents aged 14 through 17. (Baseline data available in 1991)

7.11   Reduce by 20 percent the proportion of people who possess weapons that are inappropriately stored and therefore dangerously available. (Baseline data available in 1992)

Services and Protection Objectives

7.12   Extend protocols for routinely identifying, treating, and properly referring suicide attempters, victims of sexual assault, and victims of spouse, elder, and child abuse to at least 90 percent of hospital emergency departments. (Baseline data available in 1992)

7.13   Extend to at least 45 States implementation of unexplained child death review systems. (Baseline data available in 1991)

7.14   Increase to at least 30 the number of States in which at least 50 percent of children identified as neglected or physically or sexually abused receive physical and mental evaluation with appropriate followup as a means of breaking the intergenerational cycle of abuse. (Baseline data available in 1993)

7.15   Reduce to less than 10 percent the proportion of battered women and their children turned away from emergency housing due to lack of space. (Baseline: 40 percent in 1987)

7.16   Increase to at least 50 percent the proportion of elementary and secondary schools that teach nonviolent conflict resolution skills, preferably as a part of quality school health education. (Baseline data available in 1991)

7.17   Extend coordinated, comprehensive violence prevention programs to at least 80 percent of local jurisdictions with populations over 100,000. (Baseline data available in 1993)

7.18*   Increase to 50 the number of States with officially established protocols that engage mental health, alcohol and drug, and public health authorities with corrections authorities to facilitate identification and appropriate intervention to prevent suicide by jail inmates. (Baseline data available in 1992)

8. Educational and Community-Based Programs

Health Status Objective

8.1*   Increase years of healthy life to at least 65 years. (Baseline: An estimated 62 years in 1980)

Special Population Targets

Years of Healthy Life	1980 Baseline	2000 Target
8.1a Blacks	56	60
8.1b Hispanics	62	65
8.1c People aged 65 and older	12[†]	14[†]

[†]*Years of healthy life remaining at age 65*

Note: Years of healthy life (also referred to as quality-adjusted life years) is a summary measure of health that combines mortality (quantity of life) and morbidity and disability (quality of life) into a single measure. For people aged 65 and older, active life-expectancy, a related summary measure, also will be tracked.

Risk Reduction Objective

8.2   Increase the high school graduation rate to at least 90 percent, thereby reducing risks for multiple problem behaviors and poor mental and physical health. (Baseline: 79 percent of people aged 20 through 21 had graduated from high school with a regular diploma in 1989)

Note: This objective and its target are consistent with the National Education Goal to increase high school graduation rates. The baseline estimate is a proxy. When a measure is chosen to monitor the National Education Goal, the same measure and data source will be used to track this objective.

Services and Protection Objectives

8.3   Achieve for all disadvantaged children and children with disabilities access to high quality and developmentally appropriate preschool programs that help prepare children for school, thereby improving their prospects with regard to school performance, problem behaviors, and mental and physical health. (Baseline: 47 percent of eligible children aged 4 were afforded the opportunity to enroll in Head Start in 1990)

Note: This objective and its target are consistent with the National Education Goal to increase school readiness and its objective to increase access to preschool programs for disadvantaged and disabled children. The baseline estimate is an available, but partial, proxy. When a measure is chosen to monitor this National Education Objective, the same measure and data source will be used to track this objective.

8.4   Increase to at least 75 percent the proportion of the Nation's elementary and secondary schools that provide planned and sequential kindergarten through 12th grade quality school health education. (Baseline data available in 1991)

8.5   Increase to at least 50 percent the proportion of postsecondary institutions with institutionwide health promotion programs for students, faculty, and staff. (Baseline: At least 20 percent of higher education institutions offered health promotion activities for students in 1989-90)

8.6   Increase to at least 85 percent the proportion of workplaces with 50 or more employees that offer health promotion activities for their employees, preferably as part of a comprehensive employee health promotion program. (Baseline: 65 percent of worksites with 50 or more employees offered at least one health promotion activity in 1985; 63 percent of medium and large companies had a wellness program in 1987)

8.7   Increase to at least 20 percent the proportion of hourly workers who participate regularly in employer-sponsored health promotion activities. (Baseline data available in 1992)

8.8   Increase to at least 90 percent the proportion of people aged 65 and older who had the opportunity to participate during the preceding year in at least one organized health promotion program through a senior center, lifecare facility, or other community-based setting that serves older adults. (Baseline data available in 1992)

8.9   Increase to at least 75 percent the proportion of people aged 10 and older who have discussed issues related to nutrition, physical activity, sexual behavior, tobacco, alcohol, other drugs, or safety with family members on at least one occasion during the preceding month. (Baseline data available in 1991)

Note: This objective, which supports family communication on a range of vital personal health issues, will be tracked using the National Health Interview Survey, a continuing, voluntary, national sample survey of adults who report on household characteristics including such items as illnesses, injuries, use of health services, and demographic characteristics.

8.10   Establish community health promotion programs that separately or together address at least three of the Healthy People 2000 priorities and reach at least 40 percent of each State's population. (Baseline data available in 1992)

8.11   Increase to at least 50 percent the proportion of counties that have established culturally and linguistically appropriate community health promotion programs for racial and ethnic minority populations. (Baseline data available in 1992)

Note: This objective will be tracked in counties in which a racial or ethnic group constitutes more than 10 percent of the population.

8.12   Increase to at least 90 percent the proportion of hospitals, health maintenance organizations, and large group practices that provide patient education programs, and to at least 90 percent the proportion of community hospitals that offer community health promotion programs addressing the priority health needs of their communities. (Baseline: 66 percent of 6,821 registered hospitals provided patient education services in 1987; 60 percent of 5,677 community hospitals offered community health promotion programs in 1987)

8.13   Increase to at least 75 percent the proportion of local television network affiliates in the top 20 television markets that have become partners with one or more community organizations around one of the health problems addressed by the Healthy People 2000 objectives. (Baseline data available in 1991)

8.14   Increase to at least 90 percent the proportion of people who are served by a local health department that is effectively carrying out the core functions of public health. (Baseline data available in 1992)

Note: The core functions of public health have been defined as assessment, policy development, and assurance. Local health department refers to any local component of the public health system, defined as an administrative and service unit of local or State government concerned with health and carrying some responsibility for the health of a jurisdiction smaller than a State.

9. Unintentional Injuries

Health Status Objectives

9.1 Reduce deaths caused by unintentional injuries to no more than 29.3 per 100,000 people. (Age-adjusted baseline: 34.5 per 100,000 in 1987)

Special Population Targets

Deaths Caused By Unintential Injuries (per 100,000)	1987 Baseline	2000 Target
9.1a American Indians/Alaska Natives	82.6	66.1
9.1b Black males	64.9	51.9
9.1c White males	53.6	42.9

9.2 Reduce nonfatal unintentional injuries so that hospitalizations for this condition are no more than 754 per 100,000 people. (Baseline: 887 per 100,000 in 1988)

9.3 Reduce deaths caused by motor vehicle crashes to no more than 1.9 per 100 million vehicle miles traveled and 16.8 per 100,000 people. (Baseline: 2.4 per 100 million vehicle miles traveled (VMT) and 18.8 per 100,000 people (age adjusted) in 1987)

Special Population Targets

Deaths Caused By Motor Vehicle Crashes (per 100,000)	1987 Baseline	2000 Target
9.3a Children aged 14 and younger	6.2	5.5
9.3b Youth aged 15-24	36.9	33
9.3c People aged 70 and older	22.6	20
9.3d American Indians/Alaska Natives	46.8	39.2

Type-Specific Targets

Deaths Caused By Motor Vehicle Crashes	1987 Baseline	2000 Target
9.3e Motorcyclists	40.9/100 million VMT & 1.7/100,000	33/100 million VMT & 1.5/100,000
9.3f Pedestrians	3.1/100,000	2.7/100,000

9.4 Reduce deaths from falls and fall-related injuries to no more than 2.3 per 100,000 people. (Age-adjusted baseline: 2.7 per 100,000 in 1987)

Special Population Targets

Deaths From Falls and Fall-Related Injuries (per 100,000)	1987 Baseline	2000 Target
9.4a People aged 65-84	18	14.4
9.4b People aged 85 and older	131.2	105.0
9.4c Black men aged 30-69	8	5.6

9.5 Reduce drowning deaths to no more than 1.3 per 100,000 people. (Age-adjusted baseline: 2.1 per 100,000 in 1987)

Special Population Targets

Drowning Deaths (per 100,000)	1987 Baseline	2000 Target
9.5a Children aged 4 and younger	4.2	2.3
9.5b Men aged 15-34	4.5	2.5
9.5c Black males	6.6	3.6

9.6 Reduce residential fire deaths to no more than 1.2 per 100,000 people. (Age-adjusted baseline: 1.5 per 100,000 in 1987)

Special Population Targets

Residential Fire Deaths (per 100,000)	1987 Baseline	2000 Target
9.6a Children aged 4 and younger	4.4	3.3
9.6b People aged 65 and older	4.4	3.3
9.6c Black males	5.7	4.3
9.6d Black females	3.4	2.6

Type-Specific Target

	1983 Baseline	2000 Target
9.6e Residential fire deaths caused by smoking	17%	5%

9.7 Reduce hip fractures among people aged 65 and older so that hospitalizations for this condition are no more than 607 per 100,000. (Baseline: 714 per 100,000 in 1988)

Special Population Target

Hip Fractures (per 100,000)	1988 Baseline	2000 Target
9.7a White women aged 85 and older	2,721	2,177

103

9.8 Reduce nonfatal poisoning to no more than 88 emergency department treatments per 100,000 people. (Baseline: 103 per 100,000 in 1986)

Special Population Target

Nonfatal Poisoning (per 100,000)	*1986 Baseline*	*2000 Target*
9.8a Among children aged 4 and younger	650	520

9.9 Reduce nonfatal head injuries so that hospitalizations for this condition are no more than 106 per 100,000 people. (Baseline: 125 per 100,000 in 1988)

9.10 Reduce nonfatal spinal cord injuries so that hospitalizations for this condition are no more than 5 per 100,000 people. (Baseline: 5.9 per 100,000 in 1988)

Special Population Target

Nonfatal Spinal Cord Injuries (per 100,000)	*1988 Baseline*	*2000 Target*
9.10a Males	8.9	7.1

9.11 Reduce the incidence of secondary disabilities associated with injuries of the head and spinal cord to no more than 16 and 2.6 per 100,000 people, respectively. (Baseline: 20 per 100,000 for serious head injuries and 3.2 per 100,000 for spinal cord injuries in 1986)

Note: Secondary disabilities are defined as those medical conditions secondary to traumatic head or spinal cord injury that impair independent and productive lifestyles.

Risk Reduction Objectives

9.12 Increase use of occupant protection systems, such as safety belts, inflatable safety restraints, and child safety seats, to at least 85 percent of motor vehicle occupants. (Baseline: 42 percent in 1988)

Special Population Target

Use of Occupant Protection Systems	*1988 Baseline*	*2000 Target*
9.12a Children aged 4 and younger	84%	95%

9.13 Increase use of helmets to at least 80 percent of motorcyclists and at least 50 percent of bicyclists. (Baseline: 60 percent of motorcyclists in 1988 and an estimated 8 percent of bicyclists in 1984)

Services and Protection Objectives

9.14 Extend to 50 States laws requiring safety belt and motorcycle helmet use for all ages. (Baseline: 33 States and the District of Columbia in 1989 for automobiles; 22 States, the District of Columbia, and Puerto Rico for motorcycles)

9.15 Enact in 50 States laws requiring that new handguns be designed to minimize the likelihood of discharge by children. (Baseline: 0 States in 1989)

9.16 Extend to 2,000 local jurisdictions the number whose codes address the installation of fire suppression sprinkler systems in those residences at highest risk for fires. (Baseline data available in 1991)

9.17 Increase the presence of functional smoke detectors to at least one on each habitable floor of all inhabited residential dwellings. (Baseline: 81 percent of residential dwellings in 1989)

9.18 Provide academic instruction on injury prevention and control, preferably as part of quality school health education, in at least 50 percent of public school systems (grades K through 12). (Baseline data available in 1991)

9.19* Extend requirement of the use of effective head, face, eye, and mouth protection to all organizations, agencies, and institutions sponsoring sporting and recreation events that pose risks of injury. (Baseline: Only National Collegiate Athletic Association football, hockey, and lacrosse; high school football; amateur boxing; and amateur ice hockey in 1988)

9.20 Increase to at least 30 the number of States that have design standards for signs, signals, markings, lighting, and other characteristics of the roadway environment to improve the visual stimuli and protect the safety of older drivers and pedestrians. (Baseline data available in 1992)

9.21 Increase to at least 50 percent the proportion of primary care providers who routinely provide age-appropriate counseling on safety precautions to prevent unintentional injury. (Baseline data available in 1992)

9.22 Extend to 50 States emergency medical services and trauma systems linking prehospital, hospital, and rehabilitation services in order to prevent trauma deaths and long-term disability. (Baseline: 2 States in 1987)

10. Occupational Safety and Health

Health Status Objectives

10.1 Reduce deaths from work-related injuries to no more than 4 per 100,000 full-time workers. (Baseline: Average of 6 per 100,000 during 1983-87)

Special Population Targets

Work-Related Deaths (per 100,000)	*1983-87 Average*	*2000 Target*
10.1a Mine workers	30.3	21
10.1b Construction workers	25.0	17
10.1c Transportation workers	15.2	10
10.1d Farm workers	14.0	9.5

10.2 Reduce work-related injuries resulting in medical treatment, lost time from work, or restricted work activity to no more than 6 cases per 100 full-time workers. (Baseline: 7.7 per 100 in 1987)

Special Population Targets

Work-Related Injuries (per 100)	1983-87 Average	2000 Target
10.2a Construction workers	14.9	10
10.2b Nursing and personal care workers	12.7	9
10.2c Farm workers	12.4	8
10.2d Transportation workers	8.3	6
10.2e Mine workers	8.3	6

10.3 Reduce cumulative trauma disorders to an incidence of no more than 60 cases per 100,000 full-time workers. (Baseline: 100 per 100,000 in 1987)

Special Population Targets

Cumulative Trauma Disorders (per 100,000)	1987 Baseline	2000 Target
10.3a Manufacturing industry workers	355	150
10.3b Meat product workers	3,920	2,000

10.4 Reduce occupational skin disorders or diseases to an incidence of no more than 55 per 100,000 full-time workers. (Baseline: Average of 64 per 100,000 during 1983-87)

10.5* Reduce hepatitis B infections among occupationally exposed workers to an incidence of no more than 1,250 cases. (Baseline: An estimated 6,200 cases in 1987)

Risk Reduction Objectives

10.6 Increase to at least 75 percent the proportion of worksites with 50 or more employees that mandate employee use of occupant protection systems, such as seatbelts, during all work-related motor vehicle travel. (Baseline data available in 1991)

10.7 Reduce to no more than 15 percent the proportion of workers exposed to average daily noise levels that exceed 85 dBA. (Baseline data available in 1992)

10.8 Eliminate exposures which result in workers having blood lead concentrations greater than 25 µg/dL of whole blood. (Baseline: 4,804 workers with blood lead levels above 25 µg/dL in 7 States in 1988)

10.9* Increase hepatitis B immunization levels to 90 percent among occupationally exposed workers. (Baseline data available in 1991)

Services and Protection Objectives

10.10 Implement occupational safety and health plans in 50 States for the identification, management, and prevention of leading work-related diseases and injuries within the State. (Baseline: 10 States in 1989)

10.11 Establish in 50 States exposure standards adequate to prevent the major occupational lung diseases to which their worker populations are exposed (byssinosis, asbestosis, coal workers' pneumoconiosis, and silicosis). (Baseline data available in 1991)

10.12 Increase to at least 70 percent the proportion of worksites with 50 or more employees that have implemented programs on worker health and safety. (Baseline data available in 1991)

10.13 Increase to at least 50 percent the proportion of worksites with 50 or more employees that offer back injury prevention and rehabilitation programs. (Baseline: 28.6 percent offered back care activities in 1985)

10.14 Establish in 50 States either public health or labor department programs that provide consultation and assistance to small businesses to implement safety and health programs for their employees. (Baseline data available in 1991)

10.15 Increase to at least 75 percent the proportion of primary care providers who routinely elicit occupational health exposures as a part of patient history and provide relevant counseling. (Baseline data available in 1992)

11. Environmental Health

Health Status Objectives

11.1 Reduce asthma morbidity, as measured by a reduction in asthma hospitalizations to no more than 160 per 100,000 people. (Baseline: 188 per 100,000 in 1987)

Special Population Targets

Asthma Hospitalizations (per 100,000)	1987 Baseline	2000 Target
11.1a Blacks and other nonwhites	334	265
11.1b Children	284[†]	225

†*Children aged 14 and younger*

11.2* Reduce the prevalence of serious mental retardation among school-aged children to no more than 2 per 1,000 children. (Baseline: 2.7 per 1,000 children aged 10 in 1985-88)

11.3   Reduce outbreaks of waterborne disease from infectious agents and chemical poisoning to no more than 11 per year. (Baseline: Average of 31 outbreaks per year during 1981-88)

Type-Specific Target

Average Annual Number of Waterborne Disease Outbreaks	*1981-88 Baseline*	*2000 Target*
11.3a People served by community water systems	13	6

Note: Community water systems are public or investor-owned water systems that serve large or small communities, subdivisions, or trailer parks with at least 15 service connections or 25 year-round residents.

11.4   Reduce the prevalence of blood lead levels exceeding 15 µg/dL and 25 µg/dL among children aged 6 months through 5 years to no more than 500,000 and zero, respectively. (Baseline: An estimated 3 million children had levels exceeding 15 µg/dL, and 234,000 had levels exceeding 25 µg/dL, in 1984)

Special Population Target

Prevalence of Blood Lead Levels Exceeding 15 µg/dL & 25 µg/dL	*1984 Baseline*	*2000 Target*
11.4a Inner-city low-income black children (annual family income <$6,000 in 1984 dollars)	234,900 & 36,700	75,000 & 0

Risk Reduction Objectives

11.5   Reduce human exposure to criteria air pollutants, as measured by an increase to at least 85 percent in the proportion of people who live in counties that have not exceeded any Environmental Protection Agency standard for air quality in the previous 12 months. (Baseline: 49.7 percent in 1988)

Proportion Living in Counties That Have Not Exceeded Criteria Air Pollutant Standards in 1988 for:

Ozone	53.6%
Carbon monoxide	87.8%
Nitrogen dioxide	96.6%
Sulfur dioxide	99.3%
Particulates	89.4%
Lead	99.3%
Total (any of above pollutants)	49.7%

Note: An individual living in a county that exceeds an air quality standard may not actually be exposed to unhealthy air. Of all criteria air pollutants, ozone is the most likely to have fairly uniform concentrations throughout an area. Exposure is to criteria air pollutants in ambient air. Due to weather fluctuations, multi-year averages may be the most appropriate way to monitor progress toward this objective.

11.6   Increase to at least 40 percent the proportion of homes in which homeowners/occupants have tested for radon concentrations and that have either been found to pose minimal risk or have been modified to reduce risk to health. (Baseline: Less than 5 percent of homes had been tested in 1989)

Special Population Targets

Testing and Modification As Necessary	*Baseline*	*2000 Target*
11.6a Homes with smokers and former smokers	—	50%
11.6b Homes with children	—	50%

11.7   Reduce human exposure to toxic agents by confining total pounds of toxic agents released into the air, water, and soil each year to no more than:

0.24 billion pounds of those toxic agents included on the Department of Health and Human Services list of carcinogens. (Baseline: 0.32 billion pounds in 1988)

2.6 billion pounds of those toxic agents included on the Agency for Toxic Substances and Disease Registry list of the most toxic chemicals. (Baseline: 2.62 billion pounds in 1988)

11.8   Reduce human exposure to solid waste-related water, air, and soil contamination, as measured by a reduction in average pounds of municipal solid waste produced per person each day to no more than 3.6 pounds. (Baseline: 4.0 pounds per person each day in 1988)

11.9   Increase to at least 85 percent the proportion of people who receive a supply of drinking water that meets the safe drinking water standards established by the Environmental Protection Agency. (Baseline: 74 percent of 58,099 community water systems serving approximately 80 percent of the population in 1988)

Note: Safe drinking water standards are measured using Maximum Contaminant Level (MCL) standards set by the Environmental Protection Agency which define acceptable levels of contaminants. See Objective 11.3 for definition of community water systems.

11.10   Reduce potential risks to human health from surface water, as measured by a decrease to no more than 15 percent in the proportion of assessed rivers, lakes, and estuaries that do not support beneficial uses, such as fishing and swimming. (Baseline: An estimated 25 percent of assessed rivers, lakes, and estuaries did not support designated beneficial uses in 1988)

Note: Designated beneficial uses, such as aquatic life support, contact recreation (swimming), and water supply, are designated by each State and approved by the Environmental Protection Agency. Support of beneficial use is a proxy measure of risk to human health, as many pollutants causing impaired water uses do not have human health effects (e.g., siltation, impaired fish habitat).

Services and Protection Objectives

11.11 Perform testing for lead-based paint in at least 50 percent of homes built before 1950. (Baseline data available in 1991)

11.12 Expand to at least 35 the number of States in which at least 75 percent of local jurisdictions have adopted construction standards and techniques that minimize elevated indoor radon levels in those new building areas locally determined to have elevated radon levels. (Baseline: 1 State in 1989)

Note: Since construction codes are frequently adopted by local jurisdictions rather than States, progress toward this objective also may be tracked using the proportion of cities and counties that have adopted such construction standards.

11.13 Increase to at least 30 the number of States requiring that prospective buyers be informed of the presence of lead-based paint and radon concentrations in all buildings offered for sale. (Baseline: 2 States required disclosure of lead-based paint in 1989; 1 State required disclosure of radon concentrations in 1989; 2 additional States required disclosure that radon has been found in the State and that testing is desirable in 1989)

11.14 Eliminate significant health risks from National Priority List hazardous waste sites, as measured by performance of clean-up at these sites sufficient to eliminate immediate and significant health threats as specified in health assessments completed at all sites. (Baseline: 1,082 sites were on the list in March of 1990; of these, health assessments have been conducted for approximately 1,000)

Note: The Comprehensive Environmental Response, Compensation, and Liability Act of 1980 required the Environmental Protection Agency to develop criteria for determining priorities among hazardous waste sites and to develop and maintain a list of these priority sites. The resulting list is called the National Priorities List (NPL).

11.15 Establish programs for recyclable materials and household hazardous waste in at least 75 percent of counties. (Baseline: Approximately 850 programs in 41 States collected household toxic waste in 1987; extent of recycling collections unknown)

11.16 Establish and monitor in at least 35 States plans to define and track sentinel environmental diseases. (Baseline: 0 States in 1990)

Note: Sentinel environmental diseases include lead poisoning, other heavy metal poisoning (e.g., cadmium, arsenic, and mercury), pesticide poisoning, carbon monoxide poisoning, heatstroke, hypothermia, acute chemical poisoning, methemoglobinemia, and respiratory diseases triggered by environmental factors (e.g., asthma).

12. Food and Drug Safety

Health Status Objectives

12.1 Reduce infections caused by key foodborne pathogens to incidences of no more than:

Disease (per 100,000)	1987 Baseline	2000 Target
Salmonella species	18	16
Campylobacter jejuni	50	25
Escherichia coli 0157:H7	8	4
Listeria monocytogenes	0.7	0.5

12.2 Reduce outbreaks of infections due to *Salmonella enteritidis* to fewer than 25 outbreaks yearly. (Baseline: 77 outbreaks in 1989)

Risk Reduction Objective

12.3 Increase to at least 75 percent the proportion of households in which principal food preparers routinely refrain from leaving perishable food out of the refrigerator for over 2 hours and wash cutting boards and utensils with soap after contact with raw meat and poultry. (Baseline: For refrigeration of perishable foods, 70 percent; for washing cutting boards with soap, 66 percent; and for washing utensils with soap, 55 percent, in 1988)

Services and Protection Objectives

12.4 Extend to at least 70 percent the proportion of States and territories that have implemented model food codes for institutional food operations and to at least 70 percent the proportion that have adopted the new uniform food protection code ("Unicode") that sets recommended standards for regulation of all food operations. (Baseline: For institutional food operations currently using FDA's recommended model codes, 20 percent; for the new Unicode to be released in 1991, 0 percent, in 1990)

12.5 Increase to at least 75 percent the proportion of pharmacies and other dispensers of prescription medications that use linked systems to provide alerts to potential adverse drug reactions among medications dispensed by different sources to individual patients. (Baseline data available in 1993)

12.6 Increase to at least 75 percent the proportion of primary care providers who routinely review with their patients aged 65 and older all prescribed and over-the-counter medicines taken by their patients each time a new medication is prescribed. (Baseline data available in 1992)

13. Oral Health

Health Status Objectives

13.1 Reduce dental caries (cavities) so that the proportion of children with one or more caries (in permanent or primary teeth) is no more than 35 percent among children aged 6 through 8 and no more than 60 percent among adolescents aged 15. (Baseline: 53 percent of children aged 6 through 8 in 1986-87; 78 percent of adolescents aged 15 in 1986-87)

Special Population Targets

Dental Caries Prevalence	1986-87 Baseline	2000 Target
13.1a Children aged 6-8 whose parents have less than high school education	70%	45%
13.1b American Indian/Alaska Native children aged 6-8	92%[†]	45%
	52%[‡]	
13.1c Black children aged 6-8	61%	40%
13.1d American Indian/Alaska Native adolescents aged 15	93%[‡]	70%

[†]*In primary teeth in 1983-84* [‡]*In permanent teeth in 1983-84*

13.2 Reduce untreated dental caries so that the proportion of children with untreated caries (in permanent or primary teeth) is no more than 20 percent among children aged 6 through 8 and no more than 15 percent among adolescents aged 15. (Baseline: 27 percent of children aged 6 through 8 in 1986; 23 percent of adolescents aged 15 in 1986-87)

Special Population Targets

Untreated Dental Caries:	1986-87 Baseline	2000 Target
Among Children—		
13.2a Children aged 6-8 whose parents have less than high school education	43%	30%
13.2b American Indian/Alaska Native children aged 6-8	64%[†]	35%
13.2c Black children aged 6-8	38%	25%
13.2d Hispanic children aged 6-8	36%[‡]	25%
Among Adolescents—		
13.2a Adolescents aged 15 whose parents have less than a high school education	41%	25%
13.2b American Indian/Alaska Native adolescents aged 15	84%[†]	40%
13.2c Black adolescents aged 15	38%	20%
13.2d Hispanic adolescents aged 15	31-47%[‡]	25%

[†]*1983-84 baseline* [‡]*1982-84 baseline*

13.3 Increase to at least 45 percent the proportion of people aged 35 through 44 who have never lost a permanent tooth due to dental caries or periodontal diseases. (Baseline: 31 percent of employed adults had never lost a permanent tooth for any reason in 1985-86)

Note: Never lost a permanent tooth is having 28 natural teeth exclusive of third molars.

13.4 Reduce to no more than 20 percent the proportion of people aged 65 and older who have lost all of their natural teeth. (Baseline: 36 percent in 1986)

Special Population Target

Complete Tooth Loss Prevalence	1986 Baseline	2000 Target
13.4a Low-income people (annual family income <$15,000)	46%	25%

13.5 Reduce the prevalence of gingivitis among people aged 35 through 44 to no more than 30 percent. (Baseline: 42 percent in 1985-86)

Special Population Targets

Gingivitis Prevalence	1985 Baseline	2000 Target
13.5a Low-income people (annual family income <$12,500)	50%	35%
13.5b American Indians/Alaska Natives	95%[†]	50%
13.5c Hispanics		50%
Mexican Americans	74%[‡]	
Cubans	79%[‡]	
Puerto Ricans	82%[‡]	

[†]*1983-84 baseline* [‡]*1982-84 baseline*

13.6 Reduce destructive periodontal diseases to a prevalence of no more than 15 percent among people aged 35 through 44. (Baseline: 24 percent in 1985-86)

Note: Destructive periodontal disease is one or more sites with 4 millimeters or greater loss of tooth attachment.

13.7 Reduce deaths due to cancer of the oral cavity and pharynx to no more than 10.5 per 100,000 men aged 45 through 74 and 4.1 per 100,000 women aged 45 through 74. (Baseline: 12.1 per 100,000 men and 4.1 per 100,000 women in 1987)

Risk Reduction Objectives

13.8   Increase to at least 50 percent the proportion of children who have received protective sealants on the occlusal (chewing) surfaces of permanent molar teeth. (Baseline: 11 percent of children aged 8 and 8 percent of adolescents aged 14 in 1986-87)

Note: Progress toward this objective will be monitored based on prevalence of sealants in children at age 8 and at age 14, when the majority of first and second molars, respectively, are erupted.

13.9   Increase to at least 75 percent the proportion of people served by community water systems providing optimal levels of fluoride. (Baseline: 62 percent in 1989)

Note: Optimal levels of fluoride are determined by the mean maximum daily air temperature over a 5-year period and range between 0.7 and 1.2 parts of fluoride per one million parts of water (ppm).

13.10   Increase use of professionally or self-administered topical or systemic (dietary) fluorides to at least 85 percent of people not receiving optimally fluoridated public water. (Baseline: An estimated 50 percent in 1989)

13.11*   Increase to at least 75 percent the proportion of parents and caregivers who use feeding practices that prevent baby bottle tooth decay. (Baseline data available in 1991)

Special Population Targets

Appropriate Feeding Practices	Baseline	2000 Target
13.11a Parents and caregivers with less than high school education	—	65%
13.11b American Indian/Alaska Native parents and caregivers	—	65%

Services and Protection Objectives

13.12   Increase to at least 90 percent the proportion of all children entering school programs for the first time who have received an oral health screening, referral, and followup for necessary diagnostic, preventive, and treatment services. (Baseline: 66 percent of children aged 5 visited a dentist during the previous year in 1986)

Note: School programs include Head Start, prekindergarten, kindergarten, and 1st grade.

13.13   Extend to all long-term institutional facilities the requirement that oral examinations and services be provided no later than 90 days after entry into these facilities. (Baseline: Nursing facilities receiving Medicaid or Medicare reimbursement will be required to provide for oral examinations within 90 days of patient entry beginning in 1990; baseline data unavailable for other institutions)

Note: Long-term institutional facilities include nursing homes, prisons, juvenile homes, and detention facilities.

13.14   Increase to at least 70 percent the proportion of people aged 35 and older using the oral health care system during each year. (Baseline: 54 percent in 1986)

Special Population Targets

Proportion Using Oral Health Care System During Each Year	1986 Baseline	2000 Target
13.14a Edentulous people	11%	50%
13.14b People aged 65 and older	42%	60%

13.15   Increase to at least 40 the number of States that have an effective system for recording and referring infants with cleft lips and/or palates to craniofacial anomaly teams. (Baseline: In 1988, approximately 25 States had a central recording mechanism for cleft lip and/or palate and approximately 25 States had an organized referral system to craniofacial anomaly teams)

13.16*   Extend requirement of the use of effective head, face, eye, and mouth protection to all organizations, agencies, and institutions sponsoring sporting and recreation events that pose risks of injury. (Baseline: Only National Collegiate Athletic Association football, hockey, and lacrosse; high school football; amateur boxing; and amateur ice hockey in 1988)

14. Maternal and Infant Health

Health Status Objectives

14.1 Reduce the infant mortality rate to no more than 7 per 1,000 live births. (Baseline: 10.1 per 1,000 live births in 1987)

Special Population Targets

Infant Mortality (per 1,000 live births)	1987 Baseline	2000 Target
14.1a Blacks	17.9	11
14.1b American Indians/Alaska Natives	12.5†	8.5
14.1c Puerto Ricans	12.9†	8

Type-Specific Targets

Neonatal and Postneonatal Mortality (per 1,000 live births)	1987 Baseline	2000 Target
14.1d Neonatal mortality	6.5	4.5
14.1e Neonatal mortality among blacks	11.7	7
14.1f Neonatal mortality among Puerto Ricans	8.6†	5.2
14.1g Postneonatal mortality	3.6	2.5
14.1h Postneonatal mortality among blacks	6.1	4
14.1i Postneonatal mortality among American Indians/Alaska Natives	6.5†	4
14.1j Postneonatal mortality among Puerto Ricans	4.3†	2.8

†*1984 baseline*

Note: Infant mortality is deaths of infants under 1 year; neonatal mortality is deaths of infants under 28 days; and postneonatal mortality is deaths of infants aged 28 days up to 1 year.

14.2 Reduce the fetal death rate (20 or more weeks of gestation) to no more than 5 per 1,000 live births plus fetal deaths. (Baseline: 7.6 per 1,000 live births plus fetal deaths in 1987)

Special Population Target

Fetal Deaths	1987 Baseline	2000 Target
14.2a Blacks	12.8†	7.5†

† *Per 1,000 live births plus fetal deaths*

14.3 Reduce the maternal mortality rate to no more than 3.3 per 100,000 live births. (Baseline: 6.6 per 100,000 in 1987)

Special Population Target

Maternal Mortality	1987 Baseline	2000 Target
14.3a Blacks	14.2†	5†

† *Per 100,000 live births*

Note: The objective uses the maternal mortality rate as defined by the National Center for Health Statistics. However, if other sources of maternal mortality data are used, a 50-percent reduction in maternal mortality is the intended target.

14.4 Reduce the incidence of fetal alcohol syndrome to no more than 0.12 per 1,000 live births. (Baseline: 0.22 per 1,000 live births in 1987)

Special Population Targets

Fetal Alcohol Syndrome (per 1,000 live births)	1987 Baseline	2000 Target
14.4a American Indians/Alaska Natives	4	2
14.4b Blacks	0.8	0.4

Risk Reduction Objectives

14.5 Reduce low birth weight to an incidence of no more than 5 percent of live births and very low birth weight to no more than 1 percent of live births. (Baseline: 6.9 and 1.2 percent, respectively, in 1987)

Special Population Target

	1987 Baseline	2000 Target
Low Birth Weight		
14.5a Blacks	12.7%	9%
Very Low Birth Weight		
Blacks	2.7%	2%

Note: Low birth weight is weight at birth of less than 2,500 grams; very low birth weight is weight at birth of less than 1,500 grams.

14.6 Increase to at least 85 percent the proportion of mothers who achieve the minimum recommended weight gain during their pregnancies. (Baseline: 67 percent of married women in 1980)

Note: Recommended weight gain is pregnancy weight gain recommended in the 1990 National Academy of Science's report, Nutrition During Pregnancy.

14.7 Reduce severe complications of pregnancy to no more than 15 per 100 deliveries. (Baseline: 22 hospitalizations (prior to delivery) per 100 deliveries in 1987)

Note: Severe complications of pregnancy will be measured using hospitalizations due to pregnancy-related complications.

14.8 Reduce the cesarean delivery rate to no more than 15 per 100 deliveries. (Baseline: 24.4 per 100 deliveries in 1987)

Type-Specific Targets

Cesarean Delivery (per 100 deliveries)	*1987 Baseline*	*2000 Target*
14.8a Primary (first time) cesarean delivery	17.4	12
14.8b Repeat cesarean deliveries	91.2[†]	65[†]

[†]*Among women who had a previous cesarean delivery*

14.9* Increase to at least 75 percent the proportion of mothers who breastfeed their babies in the early postpartum period and to at least 50 percent the proportion who continue breastfeeding until their babies are 5 to 6 months old. (Baseline: 54 percent at discharge from birth site and 21 percent at 5 to 6 months in 1988)

Special Population Targets

Mothers Breastfeeding Their Babies:	*1988 Baseline*	*2000 Target*
During Early Postpartum Period —		
14.9a Low-income mothers	32%	75%
14.9b Black mothers	25%	75%
14.9c Hispanic mothers	51%	75%
14.9d American Indian/Alaska Native mothers	47%	75%
At Age 5-6 Months —		
14.9a Low-income mothers	9%	50%
14.9b Black mothers	8%	50%
14.9c Hispanic mothers	16%	50%
14.9d American Indian/Alaska Native mothers	28%	50%

14.10 Increase abstinence from tobacco use by pregnant women to at least 90 percent and increase abstinence from alcohol, cocaine, and marijuana by pregnant women by at least 20 percent. (Baseline: 75 percent of pregnant women abstained from tobacco use in 1985)

Note: Data for alcohol, cocaine, and marijuana use by pregnant women will be available from the National Maternal and Infant Health Survey, CDC, in 1991.

Services and Protection Objectives

14.11 Increase to at least 90 percent the proportion of all pregnant women who receive prenatal care in the first trimester of pregnancy. (Baseline: 76 percent of live births in 1987)

Special Population Targets

Proportion of Pregnant Women Receiving Early Prenatal Care	*1987 Baseline*	*2000 Target*
14.11a Black women	61.1[†]	90[†]
14.11b American Indian/Alaska Native women	60.2[†]	90[†]
14.11c Hispanic women	61.0[†]	90[†]

[†] *Percent of live births*

14.12* Increase to at least 60 percent the proportion of primary care providers who provide age-appropriate preconception care and counseling. (Baseline data available in 1992)

14.13 Increase to at least 90 percent the proportion of women enrolled in prenatal care who are offered screening and counseling on prenatal detection of fetal abnormalities. (Baseline data available in 1991)

Note: This objective will be measured by tracking use of maternal serum alpha-fetoprotein screening tests.

14.14 Increase to at least 90 percent the proportion of pregnant women and infants who receive risk-appropriate care. (Baseline data available in 1991)

Note: This objective will be measured by tracking the proportion of very low birth weight infants (less than 1,500 grams) born in facilities covered by a neonatologist 24 hours a day.

14.15 Increase to at least 95 percent the proportion of newborns screened by State-sponsored programs for genetic disorders and other disabling conditions and to 90 percent the proportion of newborns testing positive for disease who receive appropriate treatment. (Baseline: For sickle cell anemia, with 20 States reporting, approximately 33 percent of live births screened (57 percent of black infants); for galactosemia, with 38 States reporting, approximately 70 percent of live births screened)

Note: As measured by the proportion of infants served by programs for sickle cell anemia and galactosemia. Screening programs should be appropriate for State demographic characteristics.

14.16 Increase to at least 90 percent the proportion of babies aged 18 months and younger who receive recommended primary care services at the appropriate intervals. (Baseline data available in 1992)

15. Heart Disease and Stroke

Health Status Objectives

15.1* Reduce coronary heart disease deaths to no more than 100 per 100,000 people. (Age-adjusted baseline: 135 per 100,000 in 1987)

Special Population Target

Coronary Deaths (per 100,000)	1987 Baseline	2000 Target
15.1a Blacks	163	115

15.2 Reduce stroke deaths to no more than 20 per 100,000 people. (Age-adjusted baseline: 30.3 per 100,000 in 1987)

Special Population Target

Stroke Deaths (per 100,000)	1987 Baseline	2000 Target
15.2a Blacks	51.2	27

15.3 Reverse the increase in end-stage renal disease (requiring maintenance dialysis or transplantation) to attain an incidence of no more than 13 per 100,000. (Baseline: 13.9 per 100,000 in 1987)

Special Population Target

ESRD Incidence (per 100,000)	1987 Baseline	2000 Target
15.3a Blacks	32.4	30

Risk Reduction Objectives

15.4 Increase to at least 50 percent the proportion of people with high blood pressure whose blood pressure is under control. (Baseline: 11 percent controlled among people aged 18 through 74 in 1976-80; an estimated 24 percent for people aged 18 and older in 1982-84)

Special Population Target

High Blood Pressure Control	1976-80 Baseline	1982-84 Baseline	2000 Target
15.4a Men with high blood pressure	6%	16%	40%

Note: People with high blood pressure have blood pressure equal to or greater than 140 mm Hg systolic and/or 90 mm Hg diastolic and/or take antihypertensive medication. Blood pressure control is defined as maintaining a blood pressure less than 140 mm Hg systolic and 90 mm Hg diastolic. In NHANES II and the Seven States Study, control of hypertension did not include nonpharmacologic treatment. In NHANES III, those controlling their high blood pressure without medication (e.g., through weight loss, low sodium diets, or restriction of alcohol) will be included.

15.5 Increase to at least 90 percent the proportion of people with high blood pressure who are taking action to help control their blood pressure. (Baseline: 79 percent of aware hypertensives aged 18 and older were taking action to control their blood pressure in 1985)

Special Population Targets

Taking Action to Control Blood Pressure	1985 Baseline	2000 Target
15.5a White hypertensive men aged 18-34	51%[†]	80%
15.5b Black hypertensive men aged 18-34	63%[†]	80%

[†]*Baseline for aware hypertensive men*

Note: High blood pressure is defined as blood pressure equal to or greater than 140 mm Hg systolic and/or 90 mm Hg diastolic and/or taking antihypertensive medication. Actions to control blood pressure include taking medication, dieting to lose weight, cutting down on salt, and exercising.

15.6 Reduce the mean serum cholesterol level among adults to no more than 200 mg/dL. (Baseline: 213 mg/dL among people aged 20 through 74 in 1976-80, 211 mg/dL for men and 215 mg/dL for women)

15.7 Reduce the prevalence of blood cholesterol levels of 240 mg/dL or greater to no more than 20 percent among adults. (Baseline: 27 percent for people aged 20 through 74 in 1976-80, 29 percent for women and 25 percent for men)

15.8 Increase to at least 60 percent the proportion of adults with high blood cholesterol who are aware of their condition and are taking action to reduce their blood cholesterol to recommended levels. (Baseline: 11 percent of all people aged 18 and older, and thus an estimated 30 percent of people with high blood cholesterol, were aware that their blood cholesterol level was high in 1988)

Note: "High blood cholesterol" means a level that requires diet and, if necessary, drug treatment. Actions to control high blood cholesterol include keeping medical appointments, making recommended dietary changes (e.g., reducing saturated fat, total fat, and dietary cholesterol), and, if necessary, taking prescribed medication.

15.9* Reduce dietary fat intake to an average of 30 percent of calories or less and average saturated fat intake to less than 10 percent of calories among people aged 2 and older. (Baseline: 36 percent of calories from total fat and 13 percent from saturated fat for people aged 20 through 74 in 1976-80; 36 percent and 13 percent for women aged 19 through 50 in 1985)

15.10* Reduce overweight to a prevalence of no more than 20 percent among people aged 20 and older and no more than 15 percent among adolescents aged 12 through 19. (Baseline: 26 percent for people aged 20 through 74 in 1976-80, 24 percent for men and 27 percent for women; 15 percent for adolescents aged 12 through 19 in 1976-80)

Special Population Targets

Overweight Prevalence	1976-80 Baseline[†]	2000 Target
15.10a Low-income women aged 20 and older	37%	25%
15.10b Black women aged 20 and older	44%	30%
15.10c Hispanic women aged 20 and older		25%
Mexican-American women	39%[‡]	
Cuban women	34%[‡]	
Puerto Rican women	37%[‡]	
15.10d American Indians/Alaska Natives	29-75%[§]	30%
15.10e People with disabilities	36%[+]	25%
15.10f Women with high blood pressure	50%	41%
15.10g Men with high blood pressure	39%	35%

[†]*Baseline for people aged 20-74* [‡]*1982-84 baseline for Hispanics aged 20-74*

[§]*1984-88 estimates for different tribes*

[+]*1985 baseline for people aged 20-74 who report any limitation in activity due to chronic conditions*

Note: For people aged 20 and older, overweight is defined as body mass index (BMI) equal to or greater than 27.8 for men and 27.3 for women. For adolescents, overweight is defined as BMI equal to or greater than 23.0 for males aged 12 through 14, 24.3 for males aged 15 through 17, 25.8 for males aged 18 through 19, 23.4 for females aged 12 through 14, 24.8 for females aged 15 through 17, and 25.7 for females aged 18 through 19. The values for adolescents are the age- and gender-specific 85th percentile values of the 1976-80 National Health and Nutrition Examination Survey (NHANES II), corrected for sample variation. BMI is calculated by dividing weight in kilograms by the square of height in meters. The cut points used to define overweight approximate the 120 percent of desirable body weight definition used in the 1990 objectives.

15.11* Increase to at least 30 percent the proportion of people aged 6 and older who engage regularly, preferably daily, in light to moderate physical activity for at least 30 minutes per day. (Baseline: 22 percent of people aged 18 and older were active for at least 30 minutes 5 or more times per week and 12 percent were active 7 or more times per week in 1985)

Note: Light to moderate physical activity requires sustained, rhythmic muscular movements, is at least equivalent to sustained walking, and is performed at less than 60 percent of maximum heart rate for age. Maximum heart rate equals roughly 220 beats per minute minus age. Examples may include walking, swimming, cycling, dancing, gardening and yardwork, various domestic and occupational activities, and games and other childhood pursuits.

15.12* Reduce cigarette smoking to a prevalence of no more than 15 percent among people aged 20 and older. (Baseline: 29 percent in 1987, 32 percent for men and 27 percent for women)

Special Population Targets

Cigarette Smoking Prevalence	1987 Baseline	2000 Target
15.12a People with a high school education or less aged 20 and older	34%	20%
15.12b Blue-collar workers aged 20 and older	36%	20%
15.12c Military personnel	42%[†]	20%
15.12d Blacks aged 20 and older	34%	18%
15.12e Hispanics aged 20 and older	33%[‡]	18%
15.12f American Indians/Alaska Natives	42-70%[§]	20%
15.12g Southeast Asian men	55%[+]	20%
15.12h Women of reproductive age	29%[††]	12%
15.12i Pregnant women	25%[‡‡]	10%
15.12j Women who use oral contraceptives	36%[§§]	10%

[†]*1988 baseline* [‡]*1982-84 baseline for Hispanics aged 20-74* [§]*1979-87 estimates for different tribes*
[+]*1984-88 baseline* [††]*Baseline for women aged 18-44* [‡‡]*1985 baseline* [§§]*1983 baseline*

Note: A cigarette smoker is a person who has smoked at least 100 cigarettes and currently smokes cigarettes.

Services and Protection Objectives

15.13 Increase to at least 90 percent the proportion of adults who have had their blood pressure measured within the preceding 2 years and can state whether their blood pressure was normal or high. (Baseline: 61 percent of people aged 18 and older had their blood pressure measured within the preceding 2 years and were given the systolic and diastolic values in 1985)

Note: A blood pressure measurement within the preceding 2 years refers to a measurement by a health professional or other trained observer.

15.14 Increase to at least 75 percent the proportion of adults who have had their blood cholesterol checked within the preceding 5 years. (Baseline: 59 percent of people aged 18 and older had "ever" had their cholesterol checked in 1988; 52 percent were checked "within the preceding 2 years" in 1988)

15.15 Increase to at least 75 percent the proportion of primary care providers who initiate diet and, if necessary, drug therapy at levels of blood cholesterol consistent with current management guidelines for patients with high blood cholesterol. (Baseline data available in 1991)

Note: Current treatment recommendations are outlined in detail in the Report of the Expert Panel on the Detection, Evaluation, and Treatment of High Blood Cholesterol in Adults, released by the National Cholesterol Education Program in 1987. Guidelines appropriate for children are currently being established. Treatment recommendations are likely to be refined over time. Thus, for the year 2000, "current" means whatever recommendations are then in effect.

15.16 Increase to at least 50 percent the proportion of worksites with 50 or more employees that offer high blood pressure and/or cholesterol education and control activities to their employees. (Baseline: 16.5 percent offered high blood pressure activities and 16.8 percent offered nutrition education activities in 1985)

15.17 Increase to at least 90 percent the proportion of clinical laboratories that meet the recommended accuracy standard for cholesterol measurement. (Baseline: 53 percent in 1985)

16. Cancer

Health Status Objectives

16.1* Reverse the rise in cancer deaths to achieve a rate of no more than 130 per 100,000 people. (Age-adjusted baseline: 133 per 100,000 in 1987)

Note: In its publications, the National Cancer Institute age adjusts cancer death rates to the 1970 U.S. population. Using the 1970 standard, the equivalent baseline and target values for this objective would be 171 and 175 per 100,000, respectively.

16.2* Slow the rise in lung cancer deaths to achieve a rate of no more than 42 per 100,000 people. (Age-adjusted baseline: 37.9 per 100,000 in 1987)

Note: In its publications, the National Cancer Institute age adjusts cancer death rates to the 1970 U.S. population. Using the 1970 standard, the equivalent baseline and target values for this objective would be 47.9 and 53 per 100,000, respectively.

16.3 Reduce breast cancer deaths to no more than 20.6 per 100,000 women. (Age-adjusted baseline: 22.9 per 100,000 in 1987)

Note: In its publications, the National Cancer Institute age adjusts cancer death rates to the 1970 U.S. population. Using the 1970 standard, the equivalent baseline and target values for this objective would be 27.2 and 25.2 per 100,000, respectively.

16.4 Reduce deaths from cancer of the uterine cervix to no more than 1.3 per 100,000 women. (Age-adjusted baseline: 2.8 per 100,000 in 1987)

Note: In its publications, the National Cancer Institute age adjusts cancer death rates to the 1970 U.S. population. Using the 1970 standard, the equivalent baseline and target values for this objective would be 3.2 and 1.5 per 100,000, respectively.

16.5 Reduce colorectal cancer deaths to no more than 13.2 per 100,000 people. (Age-adjusted baseline: 14.4 per 100,000 in 1987)

Note: In its publications, the National Cancer Institute age adjusts cancer death rates to the 1970 U.S. population. Using the 1970 standard, the equivalent baseline and target values for this objective would be 20.1 and 18.7 per 100,000, respectively.

Risk Reduction Objectives

16.6* Reduce cigarette smoking to a prevalence of no more than 15 percent among people aged 20 and older. (Baseline: 29 percent in 1987, 32 percent for men and 27 percent for women)

Special Population Targets

Cigarette Smoking Prevalence		1987 Baseline	2000 Target
16.6a	People with a high school education or less aged 20 and older	34%	20%
16.6b	Blue-collar workers aged 20 and older	36%	20%
16.6c	Military personnel	42%[†]	20%
16.6d	Blacks aged 20 and older	34%	18%
16.6e	Hispanics aged 20 and older	33%[‡]	18%
16.6f	American Indians/Alaska Natives	42-70%[§]	20%
16.6g	Southeast Asian men	55%[+]	20%
16.6h	Women of reproductive age	29%[††]	12%
16.6i	Pregnant women	25%[‡‡]	10%
16.6j	Women who use oral contraceptives	36%[§§]	10%

[†]*1988 baseline* [‡]*1982-84 baseline for Hispanics aged 20-74* [§]*1979-87 estimates for different tribes* [+]*1984-88 baseline* [††]*Baseline for women aged 18-44* [‡‡]*1985 baseline* [§§]*1983 baseline*

Note: A cigarette smoker is a person who has smoked at least 100 cigarettes and currently smokes cigarettes.

16.7* Reduce dietary fat intake to an average of 30 percent of calories or less and average saturated fat intake to less than 10 percent of calories among people aged 2 and older. (Baseline: 36 percent of calories from total fat and 13 percent from saturated fat for people aged 20 through 74 in 1976-80; 36 percent and 13 percent for women aged 19 through 50 in 1985)

Note: The inclusion of a saturated fat target in this objective should not be interpreted as evidence that reducing only saturated fat will reduce cancer risk. Epidemiologic and experimental animal studies suggest that the amount of fat consumed rather than the specific type of fat can influence the risk of some cancers.

16.8* Increase complex carbohydrate and fiber-containing foods in the diets of adults to 5 or more daily servings for vegetables (including legumes) and fruits, and to 6 or more daily servings for grain products. (Baseline: 2½ servings of fruits and vegetables and 3 servings of grain products for women aged 19 through 50 in 1985)

16.9 Increase to at least 60 percent the proportion of people of all ages who limit sun exposure, use sunscreens and protective clothing when exposed to sunlight, and avoid artificial sources of ultraviolet light (e.g., sun lamps, tanning booths). (Baseline data available in 1992)

Services and Protection Objectives

16.10 Increase to at least 75 percent the proportion of primary care providers who routinely counsel patients about tobacco use cessation, diet modification, and cancer screening recommendations. (Baseline: About 52 percent of internists reported counseling more than 75 percent of their smoking patients about smoking cessation in 1986)

16.11 Increase to at least 80 percent the proportion of women aged 40 and older who have ever received a clinical breast examination and a mammogram, and to at least 60 percent those aged 50 and older who have received them within the preceding 1 to 2 years. (Baseline: 36 percent of women aged 40 and older "ever" in 1987; 25 percent of women aged 50 and older "within the preceding 2 years" in 1987)

Special Population Targets

Clinical Breast Exam & Mammogram:	1987 Baseline	2000 Target
Ever Received—		
16.11a Hispanic women aged 40 and older	20%	80%
16.11b Low-income women aged 40 and older (annual family income <$10,000)	22%	80%
16.11c Women aged 40 and older with less than high school education	23%	80%
16.11d Women aged 70 and older	25%	80%
16.11e Black women aged 40 and older	28%	80%
Received Within Preceding 2 Years—		
16.11a Hispanic women aged 50 and older	18%	60%
16.11b Low-income women aged 50 and older (annual family income <$10,000)	15%	60%
16.11c Women aged 50 and older with less than high school education	16%	60%
16.11d Women aged 70 and older	18%	60%
16.11e Black women aged 50 and older	19%	60%

16.12 Increase to at least 95 percent the proportion of women aged 18 and older with uterine cervix who have ever received a Pap test, and to at least 85 percent those who received a Pap test within the preceding 1 to 3 years. (Baseline: 88 percent "ever" and 75 percent "within the preceding 3 years" in 1987)

Special Population Targets

Pap Test:	1987 Baseline	2000 Target
Ever Received—		
16.12a Hispanic women aged 18 and older	75%	95%
16.12b Women aged 70 and older	76%	95%
16.12c Women aged 18 and older with less than high school education	79%	95%
16.12d Low-income women aged 18 and older (annual family income <$10,000)	80%	95%
Received Within Preceding 3 Years—		
16.12a Hispanic women aged 18 and older	66%	80%
16.12b Women aged 70 and older	44%	70%
16.12c Women aged 18 and older with less than high school education	58%	75%
16.12d Low-income women aged 18 and older (annual family income <$10,000)	64%	80%

16.13 Increase to at least 50 percent the proportion of people aged 50 and older who have received fecal occult blood testing within the preceding 1 to 2 years, and to at least 40 percent those who have ever received proctosigmoidoscopy. (Baseline: 27 percent received fecal occult blood testing during the preceding 2 years in 1987; 25 percent had ever received proctosigmoidoscopy in 1987)

16.14 Increase to at least 40 percent the proportion of people aged 50 and older visiting a primary care provider in the preceding year who have received oral, skin, and digital rectal examinations during one such visit. (Baseline: An estimated 27 percent received a digital rectal exam during a physician visit within the preceding year in 1987)

16.15 Ensure that Pap tests meet quality standards by monitoring and certifying all cytology laboratories. (Baseline data available in 1991)

16.16 Ensure that mammograms meet quality standards by monitoring and certifying at least 80 percent of mammography facilities. (Baseline: An estimated 18 to 21 percent certified by the American College of Radiology as of June 1990)

17. Diabetes and Chronic Disabling Conditions

Health Status Objectives

Chronic Disabling Conditions

17.1* Increase years of healthy life to at least 65 years. (Baseline: An estimated 62 years in 1980)

Special Population Targets

Years of Healthy Life	1980 Baseline	2000 Target
17.1a Blacks	56	60
17.1b Hispanics	62	65
17.1c People aged 65 and older	12†	14†

†*Years of healthy life remaining at age 65*

Note: Years of healthy life (also referred to as quality-adjusted life years) is a summary measure of health that combines mortality (quantity of life) and morbidity and disability (quality of life) into a single measure. For people aged 65 and older, active life-expectancy, a related summary measure, also will be tracked.

17.2 Reduce to no more than 8 percent the proportion of people who experience a limitation in major activity due to chronic conditions. (Baseline: 9.4 percent in 1988)

Special Population Targets

Prevalence of Disability	1988 Baseline	2000 Target
17.2a Low-income people (annual family income <$10,000 in 1988)	18.9%	15%
17.2b American Indians/Alaska Natives	13.4%†	11%
17.2c Blacks	11.2%	9%

†*1983-85 baseline*

Note: Major activity refers to the usual activity for one's age-gender group whether it is working, keeping house, going to school, or living independently. Chronic conditions are defined as conditions that either (1) were first noticed 3 or more months ago, or (2) belong to a group of conditions such as heart disease and diabetes, which are considered chronic regardless of when they began.

17.3 Reduce to no more than 90 per 1,000 people the proportion of all people aged 65 and older who have difficulty in performing two or more personal care activities, thereby preserving independence. (Baseline: 111 per 1,000 in 1984-85)

Special Population Target

Difficulty Performing Self-Care Activities (per 1,000)	1984-85 Baseline	2000 Target
17.3a People aged 85 and older	371	325

Note: Personal care activities are bathing, dressing, using the toilet, getting in and out of bed or chair, and eating.

17.4 Reduce to no more than 10 percent the proportion of people with asthma who experience activity limitation. (Baseline: Average of 19.4 percent during 1986-88)

Note: Activity limitation refers to any self-reported limitation in activity attributed to asthma.

17.5 Reduce activity limitation due to chronic back conditions to a prevalence of no more than 19 per 1,000 people. (Baseline: Average of 21.9 per 1,000 during 1986-88)

Note: Chronic back conditions include intervertebral disk disorders, curvature of the back or spine, and other self-reported chronic back impairments such as permanent stiffness or deformity of the back or repeated trouble with the back. Activity limitation refers to any self-reported limitation in activity attributed to a chronic back condition.

17.6 Reduce significant hearing impairment to a prevalence of no more than 82 per 1,000 people. (Baseline: Average of 88.9 per 1,000 during 1986-88)

Special Population Target

Hearing Impairment (per 1,000)	1986-88 Baseline	2000 Target
17.6a People aged 45 and older	203	180

Note: Hearing impairment covers the range of hearing deficits from mild loss in one ear to profound loss in both ears. Generally, inability to hear sounds at levels softer (less intense) than 20 decibels (dB) constitutes abnormal hearing. Significant hearing impairment is defined as having hearing thresholds for speech poorer than 25 dB. However, for this objective, self-reported hearing impairment (i.e., deafness in one or both ears or any trouble hearing in one or both ears) will be used as a proxy measure for significant hearing impairment.

17.7 Reduce significant visual impairment to a prevalence of no more than 30 per 1,000 people. (Baseline: Average of 34.5 per 1,000 during 1986-88)

Special Population Target

Visual Impairment (per 1,000)	1986-88 Baseline	2000 Target
17.7a People aged 65 and older	87.7	70

Note: Significant visual impairment is generally defined as a permanent reduction in visual acuity and/or field of vision which is not correctable with eyeglasses or contact lenses. Severe visual impairment is defined as inability to read ordinary newsprint even with corrective lenses. For this objective, self-reported blindness in one or both eyes and other self-reported visual impairments (i.e., any trouble seeing with one or both eyes even when wearing glasses or colorblindness) will be used as a proxy measure for significant visual impairment.

17.8* Reduce the prevalence of serious mental retardation in school-aged children to no more than 2 per 1,000 children. (Baseline: 2.7 per 1,000 children aged 10 in 1985-88)

Note: Serious mental retardation is defined as an Intelligence Quotient (I.Q.) less than 50. This includes individuals defined by the American Association of Mental Retardation as profoundly retarded (I.Q. of 20 or less), severely retarded (I.Q. of 21-35), and moderately retarded (I.Q. of 36-50).

Diabetes

17.9 Reduce diabetes-related deaths to no more than 34 per 100,000 people. (Age-adjusted baseline: 38 per 100,000 in 1986)

Special Population Targets

Diabetes-Related Deaths (per 100,000)	1986 Baseline	2000 Target
17.9a Blacks	65	58
17.9b American Indians/Alaska Natives	54	48

Note: Diabetes-related deaths refer to deaths from diabetes as an underlying or contributing cause.

17.10 Reduce the most severe complications of diabetes as follows:

Complications Among People With Diabetes	1988 Baseline	2000 Target
End-stage renal disease	1.5/1,000[†]	1.4/1,000
Blindness	2.2/1,000	1.4/1,000
Lower extremity amputation	8.2/1,000[†]	4.9/1,000
Perinatal mortality[‡]	5%	2%
Major congenital malformations[‡]	8%	4%

[†]*1987 baseline*   [‡]*Among infants of women with established diabetes*

Special Population Targets for ESRD

ESRD Due to Diabetes (per 1,000)	1983-86 Baseline	2000 Target
17.10a Blacks with diabetes	2.2	2
17.10b American Indians/Alaska Natives with diabetes	2.1	1.9

Special Population Target for Amputations

Lower Extremity Amputations Due to Diabetes (per 1,000)	1984-87 Baseline	2000 Target
17.10c Blacks with diabetes	10.2	6.1

Note: End-stage renal disease (ESRD) is defined as requiring maintenance dialysis or transplantation and is limited to ESRD due to diabetes. Blindness refers to blindness due to diabetic eye disease.

17.11 Reduce diabetes to an incidence of no more than 2.5 per 1,000 people and a prevalence of no more than 25 per 1,000 people. (Baselines: 2.9 per 1,000 in 1987; 28 per 1,000 in 1987)

Special Population Targets

Prevalence of Diabetes (per 1,000)	1982-84 Baseline[†]	2000 Target
17.11a American Indians/Alaska Natives	69[‡]	62
17.11b Puerto Ricans	55	49
17.11c Mexican Americans	54	49
17.11d Cuban Americans	36	32
17.11e Blacks	36[§]	32

[†]*1982-84 baseline for people aged 20-74*

[‡]*1987 baseline for American Indians/Alaska Natives aged 15 and older*

[§]*1987 baseline for blacks of all ages*

Risk Reduction Objectives

17.12* Reduce overweight to a prevalence of no more than 20 percent among people aged 20 and older and no more than 15 percent among adolescents aged 12 through 19. (Baseline: 26 percent for people aged 20 through 74 in 1976-80, 24 percent for men and 27 percent for women; 15 percent for adolescents aged 12 through 19 in 1976-80)

Special Population Targets

Overweight Prevalence	1976-80 Baseline[†]	2000 Target
17.12a Low-income women aged 20 and older	37%	25%
17.12b Black women aged 20 and older	44%	30%
17.12c Hispanic women aged 20 and older		25%
Mexican-American women	39%[‡]	
Cuban women	34%[‡]	
Puerto Rican women	37%[‡]	
17.12d American Indians/Alaska Natives	29-75%[§]	30%
17.12e People with disabilities	36%[+]	25%
17.12f Women with high blood pressure	50%	41%
17.12g Men with high blood pressure	39%	35%

[†]*1976-80 baseline for people aged 20-74*   [‡]*1982-84 baseline for Hispanics aged 20-74*

[§]*1984-88 estimates for different tribes*

[+]*1985 baseline for people aged 20-74 who report any limitation in activity due to chronic conditions*

Note: For people aged 20 and older, overweight is defined as body mass index (BMI) equal to or greater than 27.8 for men and 27.3 for women. For adolescents, overweight is defined as BMI equal to or greater than 23.0 for males aged 12 through 14, 24.3 for males aged 15 through 17, 25.8 for males aged 18 through 19, 23.4 for females aged 12 through 14, 24.8 for females aged 15 through 17, and 25.7 for females aged 18 through 19. The values for adolescents are the age- and gender-specific 85th percentile values of the 1976-80 National Health and Nutrition Examination Survey (NHANES II), corrected for sample variation. BMI is calculated by dividing weight in kilograms by the square of height in meters. The cut points used to define overweight approximate the 120 percent of desirable body weight definition used in the 1990 objectives.

17.13* Increase to at least 30 percent the proportion of people aged 6 and older who engage regularly, preferably daily, in light to moderate physical activity for at least 30 minutes per day. (Baseline: 22 percent of people aged 18 and older were active for at least 30 minutes 5 or more times per week and 12 percent were active 7 or more times per week in 1985)

Note: Light to moderate physical activity requires sustained, rhythmic muscular movements, is at least equivalent to sustained walking, and is performed at less than 60 percent of maximum heart rate for age. Maximum heart rate equals roughly 220 beats per minute minus age. Examples may include walking, swimming, cycling, dancing, gardening and yardwork, various domestic and occupational activities, and games and other childhood pursuits.

Services and Protection Objectives

17.14 Increase to at least 40 percent the proportion of people with chronic and disabling conditions who receive formal patient education including information about community and self-help resources as an integral part of the management of their condition. (Baseline data available in 1991)

Type-Specific Targets

Patient Education	1983-84 Baseline	2000 Target
17.14a People with diabetes	32% (classes)	75%
	68% (counseling)	
17.14b People with asthma	—	50%

17.15 Increase to at least 80 percent the proportion of providers of primary care for children who routinely refer or screen infants and children for impairments of vision, hearing, speech and language, and assess other developmental milestones as part of well-child care. (Baseline data available in 1992)

17.16 Reduce the average age at which children with significant hearing impairment are identified to no more than 12 months. (Baseline: Estimated as 24 to 30 months in 1988)

17.17 Increase to at least 60 percent the proportion of providers of primary care for older adults who routinely evaluate people aged 65 and older for urinary incontinence and impairments of vision, hearing, cognition, and functional status. (Baseline data available in 1992)

17.18 Increase to at least 90 percent the proportion of perimenopausal women who have been counseled about the benefits and risks of estrogen replacement therapy (combined with progestin, when appropriate) for prevention of osteoporosis. (Baseline data available in 1991)

17.19 Increase to at least 75 percent the proportion of worksites with 50 or more employees that have a voluntarily established policy or program for the hiring of people with disabilities. (Baseline: 37 percent of medium and large companies in 1986)

Note: Voluntarily established policies and programs for the hiring of people with disabilities are encouraged for worksites of all sizes. This objective is limited to worksites with 50 or more employees for tracking purposes.

17.20   Increase to 50 the number of States that have service systems for children with or at risk of chronic and disabling conditions, as required by Public Law 101-239. (Baseline data available in 1991)

> *Note: Children with or at risk of chronic and disabling conditions, often referred to as children with special health care needs, include children with psychosocial as well as physical problems. This population encompasses children with a wide variety of actual or potential disabling conditions, including children with or at risk for cerebral palsy, mental retardation, sensory deprivation, developmental disabilities, spina bifida, hemophilia, other genetic disorders, and health-related educational and behavioral problems. Service systems for such children are organized networks of comprehensive, community-based, coordinated, and family-centered services.*

18. HIV Infection

Health Status Objectives

18.1   Confine annual incidence of diagnosed AIDS cases to no more than 98,000 cases. (Baseline: An estimated 44,000 to 50,000 diagnosed cases in 1989)

Special Population Targets

Diagnosed AIDS Cases	1989 Baseline	2000 Target
18.1a Gay and bisexual men	26,000-28,000	48,000
18.1b Blacks	14,000-15,000	37,000
18.1c Hispanics	7,000-8,000	18,000

Note: Targets for this objective are equal to upper bound estimates of the incidence of diagnosed AIDS cases projected for 1993.

18.2   Confine the prevalence of HIV infection to no more than 800 per 100,000 people. (Baseline: An estimated 400 per 100,000 in 1989)

Special Population Targets

Estimated Prevalence of HIV Infection (per 100,000)	1989 Baseline	2000 Target
18.2a Homosexual men	2,000-42,000[†]	20,000
18.2b Intravenous drug abusers	30,000-40,000[‡]	40,000
18.2c Women giving birth to live-born infants	150	100

[†]*Per 100,000 homosexual men aged 15 through 24 based on men tested in selected sexually transmitted disease clinics in unlinked surveys; most studies find HIV prevalence of between 2,000 and 21,000 per 100,000*

[‡]*Per 100,000 intravenous drug abusers aged 15 through 24 in the New York city vicinity; in areas other than major metropolitan centers, infection rates in people entering selected drug treatment programs tested in unlinked surveys are often under 500 per 100,000*

Risk Reduction Objectives

18.3*   Reduce the proportion of adolescents who have engaged in sexual intercourse to no more than 15 percent by age 15 and no more than 40 percent by age 17. (Baseline: 27 percent of girls and 33 percent of boys by age 15; 50 percent of girls and 66 percent of boys by age 17; reported in 1988)

18.4*   Increase to at least 50 percent the proportion of sexually active, unmarried people who used a condom at last sexual intercourse. (Baseline: 19 percent of sexually active, unmarried women aged 15 through 44 reported that their partners used a condom at last sexual intercourse in 1988)

Special Population Targets

Use of Condoms	1988 Baseline	2000 Target
18.4a Sexually active young women aged 15-19 (by their partners)	26%	60%
18.4b Sexually active young men aged 15-19	57%	75%
18.4c Intravenous drug abusers	—	60%

Note: Strategies to achieve this objective must be undertaken sensitively to avoid indirectly encouraging or condoning sexual activity among teens who are not yet sexually active.

18.5   Increase to at least 50 percent the estimated proportion of all intravenous drug abusers who are in drug abuse treatment programs. (Baseline: An estimated 11 percent of opiate abusers were in treatment in 1989)

18.6   Increase to at least 50 percent the estimated proportion of intravenous drug abusers not in treatment who use only uncontaminated drug paraphernalia ("works"). (Baseline: 25 to 35 percent of opiate abusers in 1989)

18.7   Reduce to no more than 1 per 250,000 units of blood and blood components the risk of transfusion-transmitted HIV infection. (Baseline: 1 per 40,000 to 150,000 units in 1989)

Services and Protection Objectives

18.8   Increase to at least 80 percent the proportion of HIV-infected people who have been tested for HIV infection. (Baseline: An estimated 15 percent of approximately 1,000,000 HIV-infected people had been tested at publicly funded clinics, in 1989)

18.9*   Increase to at least 75 percent the proportion of primary care and mental health care providers who provide age-appropriate counseling on the prevention of HIV and other sexually transmitted diseases. (Baseline: 10 percent of physicians reported that they regularly assessed the sexual behaviors of their patients in 1987)

Special Population Target

Counseling on HIV and STD Prevention	1987 Baseline	2000 Target
18.9a Providers practicing in high incidence areas	—	90%

Note: Primary care providers include physicians, nurses, nurse practitioners, and physician assistants. Areas of high AIDS and sexually transmitted disease incidence are cities and States with incidence rates of AIDS cases, HIV seroprevalence, gonorrhea, or syphilis that are at least 25 percent above the national average.

18.10   Increase to at least 95 percent the proportion of schools that have age-appropriate HIV education curricula for students in 4th through 12th grade, preferably as part of quality school health education. (Baseline: 66 percent of school districts required HIV education but only 5 percent required HIV education in each year for 7th through 12th grade in 1989)

Note: Strategies to achieve this objective must be undertaken sensitively to avoid indirectly encouraging or condoning sexual activity among teens who are not yet sexually active.

18.11   Provide HIV education for students and staff in at least 90 percent of colleges and universities. (Baseline data available in 1995)

18.12   Increase to at least 90 percent the proportion of cities with populations over 100,000 that have outreach programs to contact drug abusers (particularly intravenous drug abusers) to deliver HIV risk reduction messages. (Baseline data available in 1995)

Note: HIV risk reduction messages include messages about reducing or eliminating drug use, entering drug treatment, disinfection of injection equipment if still injecting drugs, and safer sex practices.

18.13*   Increase to at least 50 percent the proportion of family planning clinics, maternal and child health clinics, sexually transmitted disease clinics, tuberculosis clinics, drug treatment centers, and primary care clinics that screen, diagnose, treat, counsel, and provide (or refer for) partner notification services for HIV infection and bacterial sexually transmitted diseases (gonorrhea, syphilis, and chlamydia). (Baseline: 40 percent of family planning clinics for bacterial sexually transmitted diseases in 1989)

18.14   Extend to all facilities where workers are at risk for occupational transmission of HIV regulations to protect workers from exposure to bloodborne infections, including HIV infection. (Baseline data available in 1992)

Note: The Occupational Safety and Health Administration (OSHA) is expected to issue regulations requiring worker protection from exposure to bloodborne infections, including HIV, during 1991. Implementation of the OSHA regulations would satisfy this objective.

19. Sexually Transmitted Diseases

Health Status Objectives

19.1   Reduce gonorrhea to an incidence of no more than 225 cases per 100,000 people. (Baseline: 300 per 100,000 in 1989)

Special Population Targets

Gonorrhea Incidence (per 100,000)	1989 Baseline	2000 Target
19.1a Blacks	1,990	1,300
19.1b Adolescents aged 15-19	1,123	750
19.1c Women aged 15-44	501	290

19.2   Reduce *Chlamydia trachomatis* infections, as measured by a decrease in the incidence of nongonococcal urethritis to no more than 170 cases per 100,000 people. (Baseline: 215 per 100,000 in 1988)

19.3   Reduce primary and secondary syphilis to an incidence of no more than 10 cases per 100,000 people. (Baseline: 18.1 per 100,000 in 1989)

Special Population Target

Primary and Secondary Syphilis Incidence (per 100,000)	1989 Baseline	2000 Target
19.3a Blacks	118	65

19.4   Reduce congenital syphilis to an incidence of no more than 50 cases per 100,000 live births. (Baseline: 100 per 100,000 live births in 1989)

19.5   Reduce genital herpes and genital warts, as measured by a reduction to 142,000 and 385,000, respectively, in the annual number of first-time consultations with a physician for the conditions. (Baseline: 167,000 and 451,000 in 1988)

19.6   Reduce the incidence of pelvic inflammatory disease, as measured by a reduction in hospitalizations for pelvic inflammatory disease to no more than 250 per 100,000 women aged 15 through 44. (Baseline: 311 per 100,000 in 1988)

19.7*   Reduce sexually transmitted hepatitis B infection to no more than 30,500 cases. (Baseline: 58,300 cases in 1988)

19.8   Reduce the rate of repeat gonorrhea infection to no more than 15 percent within the previous year. (Baseline: 20 percent in 1988)

Note: As measured by a reduction in the proportion of gonorrhea patients who, within the previous year, were treated for a separate case of gonorrhea.

Risk Reduction Objectives

19.9* Reduce the proportion of adolescents who have engaged in sexual intercourse to no more than 15 percent by age 15 and no more than 40 percent by age 17. (Baseline: 27 percent of girls and 33 percent of boys by age 15; 50 percent of girls and 66 percent of boys by age 17; reported in 1988)

19.10* Increase to at least 50 percent the proportion of sexually active, unmarried people who used a condom at last sexual intercourse. (Baseline: 19 percent of sexually active, unmarried women aged 15 through 44 reported that their partners used a condom at last sexual intercourse in 1988)

Special Population Targets

Use of Condoms	1988 Baseline	2000 Target
19.10a Sexually active young women aged 15-19 (by their partners)	25%	60%
19.10b Sexually active young men aged 15-19	57%	75%
19.10c Intravenous drug abusers	—	60%

Note: Strategies to achieve this objective must be undertaken sensitively to avoid indirectly encouraging or condoning sexual activity among teens who are not yet sexually active.

Services and Protection Objectives

19.11* Increase to at least 50 percent the proportion of family planning clinics, maternal and child health clinics, sexually transmitted disease clinics, tuberculosis clinics, drug treatment centers, and primary care clinics that screen, diagnose, treat, counsel, and provide (or refer for) partner notification services for HIV infection and bacterial sexually transmitted diseases (gonorrhea, syphilis, and chlamydia). (Baseline: 40 percent of family planning clinics for bacterial sexually transmitted diseases in 1989)

19.12 Include instruction in sexually transmitted disease transmission prevention in the curricula of all middle and secondary schools, preferably as part of quality school health education. (Baseline: 95 percent of schools reported offering at least one class on sexually transmitted diseases as part of their standard curricula in 1988)

Note: Strategies to achieve this objective must be undertaken sensitively to avoid indirectly encouraging or condoning sexual activity among teens who are not yet sexually active.

19.13 Increase to at least 90 percent the proportion of primary care providers treating patients with sexually transmitted diseases who correctly manage cases, as measured by their use of appropriate types and amounts of therapy. (Baseline: 70 percent in 1988)

19.14* Increase to at least 75 percent the proportion of primary care and mental health care providers who provide age-appropriate counseling on the prevention of HIV and other sexually transmitted diseases. (Baseline: 10 percent of physicians reported that they regularly assessed the sexual behaviors of their patients in 1987)

Special Population Target

Counseling on HIV and STD Prevention	1987 Baseline	2000 Target
19.14a Providers practicing in high incidence areas	—	90%

Note: Primary care providers include physicians, nurses, nurse practitioners, and physician assistants. Areas of high AIDS and sexually transmitted disease incidence are cities and States with incidence rates of AIDS cases, HIV seroprevalence, gonorrhea, or syphilis that are at least 25 percent above the national average.

19.15 Increase to at least 50 percent the proportion of all patients with bacterial sexually transmitted diseases (gonorrhea, syphilis, and chlamydia) who are offered provider referral services. (Baseline: 20 percent of those treated in sexually transmitted disease clinics in 1988)

Note: Provider referral (previously called contact tracing) is the process whereby health department personnel directly notify the sexual partners of infected individuals of their exposure to an infected individual.

20. Immunization and Infectious Diseases

Health Status Objectives

20.1 Reduce indigenous cases of vaccine-preventable diseases as follows:

Disease	1988 Baseline	2000 Target
Diphtheria among people aged 25 and younger	1	0
Tetanus among people aged 25 and younger	3	0
Polio (wild-type virus)	0	0
Measles	3,058	0
Rubella	225	0
Congenital Rubella Syndrome	6	0
Mumps	4,866	500
Pertussis	3,450	1,000

20.2 Reduce epidemic-related pneumonia and influenza deaths among people aged 65 and older to no more than 7.3 per 100,000. (Baseline: Average of 9.1 per 100,000 during 1980 through 1987)

Note: Epidemic-related pneumonia and influenza deaths are those that occur above and beyond the normal yearly fluctuations of mortality. Because of the extreme variability in epidemic-related deaths from year to year, the target is a 3-year average.

20.3* Reduce viral hepatitis as follows:

(Per 100,000)	1987 Baseline	2000 Target
Hepatitis B (HBV)	63.5	40
Hepatitis A	31	23
Hepatitis C	18.3	13.7

Special Population Targets for HBV

HBV Cases	1987 Estimated Baseline	2000 Target
20.3a Intravenous drug abusers	30,000	22,500
20.3b Heterosexually active people	33,000	22,000
20.3c Homosexual men	25,300	8,500
20.3d Children of Asians/Pacific Islanders	8,900	1,800
20.3e Occupationally exposed workers	6,200	1,250
20.3f Infants	3,500	550 new carriers
20.3g Alaska Natives	15	1

20.4 Reduce tuberculosis to an incidence of no more than 3.5 cases per 100,000 people. (Baseline: 9.1 per 100,000 in 1988)

Special Population Targets

Tuberculosis Cases (per 100,000)	1988 Baseline	2000 Target
20.4a Asians/Pacific Islanders	36.3	15
20.4b Blacks	28.3	10
20.4c Hispanics	18.3	5
20.4d American Indians/Alaska Natives	18.1	5

20.5 Reduce by at least 10 percent the incidence of surgical wound infections and nosocomial infections in intensive care patients. (Baseline data available in late 1990)

20.6 Reduce selected illness among international travelers as follows:

Incidence	1987 Baseline	2000 Target
Typhoid fever	280	140
Hepatitis A	1,280	640
Malaria	2,000	1,000

20.7 Reduce bacterial meningitis to no more than 4.7 cases per 100,000 people. (Baseline: 6.3 per 100,000 in 1986)

Special Population Target

Bacterial Meningitis Cases (per 100,000)	1987 Baseline	2000 Target
20.7a Alaska Natives	33	8

20.8 Reduce infectious diarrhea by at least 25 percent among children in licensed child care centers and children in programs that provide an Individualized Education Program (IEP) or Individualized Health Plan (IHP). (Baseline data available in 1992)

20.9 Reduce acute middle ear infections among children aged 4 and younger, as measured by days of restricted activity or school absenteeism, to no more than 105 days per 100 children. (Baseline: 131 days per 100 children in 1987)

20.10 Reduce pneumonia-related days of restricted activity as follows:

	1987 Baseline	2000 Target
People aged 65 and older (per 100 people)	48 days	38 days
Children aged 4 and younger (per 100 children)	27 days	24 days

Risk Reduction Objectives

20.11 Increase immunization levels as follows:

Basic immunization series among children under age 2: at least 90 percent. (Baseline: 70-80 percent estimated in 1989)

Basic immunization series among children in licensed child care facilities and kindergarten through post-secondary education institutions: at least 95 percent. (Baseline: For licensed child care, 94 percent; 97 percent for children entering school for the 1987-1988 school year; and for post-secondary institutions, baseline data available in 1992)

Pneumococcal pneumonia and influenza immunization among institutionalized chronically ill or older people: at least 80 percent. (Baseline data available in 1992)

Pneumococcal pneumonia and influenza immunization among noninstitutionalized, high-risk populations, as defined by the Immunization Practices Advisory Committee: at least 60 percent. (Baseline: 10 percent estimated for pneumococcal vaccine and 20 percent for influenza vaccine in 1985)

Hepatitis B immunization among high-risk populations, including infants of surface antigen-positive mothers to at least 90 percent; occupationally exposed workers to at least 90 percent; IV-drug users in drug treatment programs to at least 50 percent; and homosexual men to at least 50 percent. (Baseline data available in 1992)

20.12 Reduce postexposure rabies treatments to no more than 9,000 per year. (Baseline: 18,000 estimated treatments in 1987)

Services and Protection Objectives

20.13 Expand immunization laws for schools, preschools, and day care settings to all States for all antigens. (Baseline: 9 States and the District of Columbia in 1990)

20.14 Increase to at least 90 percent the proportion of primary care providers who provide information and counseling about immunizations and offer immunizations as appropriate for their patients. (Baseline data available in 1992)

20.15 Improve the financing and delivery of immunizations for children and adults so that virtually no American has a financial barrier to receiving recommended immunizations. (Baseline: Financial coverage for immunizations was included in 45 percent of employment-based insurance plans with conventional insurance plans; 62 percent with Preferred Provider Organization plans; and 98 percent with Health Maintenance Organization plans in 1989; Medicaid covered basic immunizations for eligible children and Medicare covered pneumococcal immunization for eligible older adults in 1990)

20.16 Increase to at least 90 percent the proportion of public health departments that provide adult immunization for influenza, pneumococcal disease, hepatitis B, tetanus, and diphtheria. (Baseline data available in 1991)

20.17 Increase to at least 90 percent the proportion of local health departments that have ongoing programs for actively identifying cases of tuberculosis and latent infection in populations at high risk for tuberculosis. (Baseline data available in 1991)

Note: Local health department refers to any local component of the public health system, defined as an administrative and service unit of local or State government concerned with health and carrying some responsibility for the health of a jurisdiction smaller than a State.

20.18 Increase to at least 85 percent the proportion of people found to have tuberculosis infection who completed courses of preventive therapy. (Baseline: 89 health departments reported that 66.3 percent of 95,201 persons placed on preventive therapy completed their treatment in 1987)

20.19 Increase to at least 85 percent the proportion of tertiary care hospital laboratories and to at least 50 percent the proportion of secondary care hospital and health maintenance organization laboratories possessing technologies for rapid viral diagnosis of influenza. (Baseline data available in 1992)

21. Clinical Preventive Services

Health Status Objective

21.1* Increase years of healthy life to at least 65 years. (Baseline: An estimated 62 years in 1980)

Special Population Targets

Years of Healthy Life	*1980 Baseline*	*2000 Target*
21.1a Blacks	56	60
21.1b Hispanics	62	65
21.1c People aged 65 and older	12[†]	14[†]

[†]*Years of healthy life remaining at age 65*

Note: Years of healthy life (also referred to as quality-adjusted life years) is a summary measure of health that combines mortality (quantity of life) and morbidity and disability (quality of life) into a single measure. For people aged 65 and older, active life-expectancy, a related summary measure, also will be tracked.

Risk Reduction Objective

21.2 Increase to at least 50 percent the proportion of people who have received, as a minimum within the appropriate interval, all of the screening and immunization services and at least one of the counseling services appropriate for their age and gender as recommended by the U.S. Preventive Services Task Force. (Baseline data available in 1991)

Special Population Targets

Receipt of Recommended Services	*Baseline*	*2000 Target*
21.2a Infants up to 24 months	—	90%
21.2b Children aged 2-12	—	80%
21.2c Adolescents aged 13-18	—	50%
21.2d Adults aged 19-39	—	40%
21.2e Adults aged 40-64	—	40%
21.2f Adults aged 65 and older	—	40%
21.2g Low-income people	—	50%
21.2h Blacks	—	50%
21.2i Hispanics	—	50%
21.2j Asians/Pacific Islanders	—	50%
21.2k American Indians/Alaska Natives	—	70%
21.2l People with disabilities	—	80%

Services and Protection Objectives

21.3　Increase to at least 95 percent the proportion of people who have a specific source of ongoing primary care for coordination of their preventive and episodic health care. (Baseline: Less than 82 percent in 1986, as 18 percent reported having no physician, clinic, or hospital as a regular source of care)

Special Population Targets

Percentage With Source of Care	1986 Baseline	2000 Target
21.3a　Hispanics	70%	95%
21.3b　Blacks	80%	95%
21.3c　Low-income people	80%	95%

21.4　Improve financing and delivery of clinical preventive services so that virtually no American has a financial barrier to receiving, at a minimum, the screening, counseling, and immunization services recommended by the U.S. Preventive Services Task Force. (Baseline data available in 1992)

21.5　Assure that at least 90 percent of people for whom primary care services are provided directly by publicly funded programs are offered, at a minimum, the screening, counseling, and immunization services recommended by the U.S. Preventive Services Task Force. (Baseline data available in 1992)

Note: Publicly funded programs that provide primary care services directly include federally funded programs such as the Maternal and Child Health Program, Community and Migrant Health Centers, and the Indian Health Service as well as primary care service settings funded by State and local governments. This objective does not include services covered indirectly through the Medicare and Medicaid programs.

21.6　Increase to at least 50 percent the proportion of primary care providers who provide their patients with the screening, counseling, and immunization services recommended by the U.S. Preventive Services Task Force. (Baseline data available in 1992)

21.7　Increase to at least 90 percent the proportion of people who are served by a local health department that assesses and assures access to essential clinical preventive services. (Baseline data available in 1992)

Note: Local health department refers to any local component of the public health system, defined as an administrative and service unit of local or State government concerned with health and carrying some responsibility for the health of a jurisdiction smaller than a State.

21.8　Increase the proportion of all degrees in the health professions and allied and associated health profession fields awarded to members of underrepresented racial and ethnic minority groups as follows:

Degrees Awarded To:	1985-86 Baseline	2000 Target
Blacks	5%	8%
Hispanics	3%	6.4%
American Indians/Alaska Natives	0.3%	0.6%

Note: Underrepresented minorities are those groups consistently below parity in most health profession schools— blacks, Hispanics, and American Indians and Alaska Natives.

22.　Surveillance and Data Systems

Objectives

22.1　Develop a set of health status indicators appropriate for Federal, State, and local health agencies and establish use of the set in at least 40 States. (Baseline: No such set exists in 1990)

22.2　Identify, and create where necessary, national data sources to measure progress toward each of the year 2000 national health objectives. (Baseline: 77 percent of the objectives have baseline data in 1990)

Type-Specific Target

	1989 Baseline	2000 Target
22.2a　State level data for at least two-thirds of the objectives	23 States[†]	35 States

[†]*Measured using the 1989 Draft Year 2000 National Health Objectives*

22.3　Develop and disseminate among Federal, State, and local agencies procedures for collecting comparable data for each of the year 2000 national health objectives and incorporate these into Public Health Service data collection systems. (Baseline: Although such surveys as the National Health Interview Survey may serve as a model, widely accepted procedures do not exist in 1990)

22.4　Develop and implement a national process to identify significant gaps in the Nation's disease prevention and health promotion data, including data for racial and ethnic minorities, people with low incomes, and people with disabilities, and establish mechanisms to meet these needs. (Baseline: No such process exists in 1990)

Note: Disease prevention and health promotion data includes disease status, risk factors, and services receipt data. Public health problems include such issue areas as HIV infection, domestic violence, mental health, environmental health, occupational health, and disabling conditions.

22.5   Implement in all States periodic analysis and publication of data needed to measure progress toward objectives for at least 10 of the priority areas of the national health objectives. (Baseline: 20 States reported that they disseminate the analyses they use to assess State progress toward the health objectives to the public and to health professionals in 1989)

Type-Specific Target

	1989 Baseline	*2000 Target*
22.5a Periodic analysis and publication of State progress toward the national objectives for each racial or ethnic group that makes up at least 10 percent of the State population	—	25 States

Note: Periodic is at least once every 3 years. Objectives include, at a minimum, one from each objectives category: health status, risk reduction, and services and protection.

22.6   Expand in all States systems for the transfer of health information related to the national health objectives among Federal, State, and local agencies. (Baseline: 30 States reported that they have some capability for transfer of health data, tables, graphs, and maps to Federal, State, and local agencies that collect and analyze data in 1989)

Note: Information related to the national health objectives includes State and national level baseline data, disease prevention/health promotion evaluation results, and data generated to measure progress.

22.7   Achieve timely release of national surveillance and survey data needed by health professionals and agencies to measure progress toward the national health objectives. (Baseline data available in 1993)

Note: Timely release (publication of provisional or final data or public use data tapes) should be based on the use of the data, but is at least within one year of the end of data collection.

Age-Related Objectives

*Reduce the death rate for children by 15 percent to no more than 28 per 100,000 children aged 1 through 14, and for infants by approximately 30 percent to no more than 7 per 1,000 live births. (Baseline: 33 per 100,000 for children in 1987 and 10.1 per 1,000 live births for infants in 1987)

Reduce the death rate for adolescents and young adults by 15 percent to no more than 85 per 100,000 people aged 15 through 24. (Baseline: 99.4 per 100,000 in 1987)

Reduce the death rate for adults by 20 percent to no more than 340 per 100,000 people aged 25 through 64. (Baseline: 423 per 100,000 in 1987)

*Reduce to no more than 90 per 1,000 people the proportion of all people aged 65 and older who have difficulty in performing two or more personal care activities (a reduction of about 19 percent), thereby preserving independence. (Baseline: 111 per 1,000 in 1984-85)

B. Contributors to *Healthy People 2000*

Healthy People 2000: National Health Promotion and Disease Prevention Objectives is the product of a national effort that has involved professionals and citizens, private organizations and public agencies from every part of the Nation. Work on the report began in 1987 with the formation of the Healthy People 2000 Consortium and the convening of public hearings across the country. Testimony from the public hearings became the primary resource material for working groups of professionals to use in crafting the health objectives themselves. After extensive public review and comment, involving more than 10,000 people, the objectives were refined and revised to produce the report.

Preparation of the report was sponsored by the U.S. Public Health Service, through a project coordinated by the Deputy Assistant Secretary for Health (Disease Prevention and Health Promotion). Project management was facilitated by the work of the PHS Steering Committee on the Healthy People 2000 Objectives; the Committee on Health Objectives for the Year 2000, Institute of Medicine, National Academy of Sciences; and the Secretary's Council on Health Promotion and Disease Prevention. Principal staff and editorial responsibility for the project was carried out by James A. Harrell, Lynn M. Artz, Ashley Files, and David Baker. Other staff from the Office of Disease Prevention and Health Promotion helping in the coordination and development of the overall project included Barbara Anderson, John Bailar, Amber Barnato, Sandra Buesking, Mary Jo Deering, Christopher DeGraw, Olga Emgushov, Martha G. Frazier, Toni M. Goodwin, Linda M. Harris, Douglas B. Kamerow, Thomas Kim, Loretta M. Logan, Patricia Lynch, Caroline McNeil, Linda D. Meyers, Diane Rittenhouse, Marilyn K. Schulenberg, Sara L. White, Jennifer Woods, Christina Wypijewski, Michael Yao, and Daniel Yarano.

While it is not possible to recognize herein all those citizens and officials who made contributions to *Healthy People 2000*, their efforts were central to development of the final product.

Public Health Service Office Directors and Agency Heads

James O. Mason, Assistant Secretary for Health, Washington, DC

Audrey F. Manley, Deputy Assistant Secretary for Health, Washington, DC

Antonia C. Novello, Surgeon General, Washington, DC

Paul B. Simmons, Deputy Assistant Secretary for Health (Communications), Washington, DC

J. Michael McGinnis, Deputy Assistant Secretary for Health (Disease Prevention and Health Promotion), Washington, DC

Samuel Lin, Deputy Assistant Secretary for Health (Intergovernmental Affairs), Rockville, MD

John D. Mahoney, Acting Deputy Assistant Secretary for Health (Operations), Washington, DC

Nabers Cabaniss, Deputy Assistant Secretary for Health (Population Affairs), Washington, DC

James M. Friedman, Acting Deputy Assistant Secretary for Health (Planning and Evaluation), Washington, DC

Frank E. Young, Deputy Assistant Secretary for Health (Science and Environment), Washington, DC

James R. Allen, Director, National AIDS Program Office, Washington, DC

Harold P. Thompson, Director, Office of International Health, Rockville, MD

William A. Robinson, Director, Office of Minority Health, Washington, DC

Wilmer D. Mizell, Executive Director, President's Council on Physical Fitness and Sports, Washington, DC

Agency Heads

J. Jarrett Clinton, Acting Administrator, Agency for Health Care Policy and Research, Rockville, MD

Frederick K. Goodwin, Administrator, Alcohol, Drug Abuse, and Mental Health Administration, Rockville, MD

William L. Roper, Director, Centers for Disease Control, and Administrator, Agency for Toxic Substances and Disease Registry, Atlanta, GA

James S. Benson, Acting Commissioner of Food and Drugs, Food and Drug Administration, Rockville, MD

Robert G. Harmon, Administrator, Health Resources and Services Administration, Rockville, MD

Everett R. Rhoades, Director, Indian Health Service, Rockville, MD

William F. Raub, Acting Director, National Institutes of Health, Bethesda, MD

Public Health Service Steering Committee on the Healthy People 2000 Objectives

PHS Members, by Agency

James A. Harrell, *Chair*, Office of Disease Prevention and Health Promotion, Washington, DC

Martha F. Katz, *Vice-Chair*, Office of Program Planning and Evaluation, Centers for Disease Control, Atlanta, GA

Elaine M. Johnson, Alcohol, Drug Abuse, and Mental Health Administration, Rockville, MD

Mary A. Jansen (alternate), Alcohol, Drug Abuse, and Mental Health Administration, Rockville, MD

Dennis D. Tolsma (alternate), Centers for Disease Control, Atlanta, GA

Ronald W. Wilson, National Center for Health Statistics, Centers for Disease Control, Hyattsville, MD

Ronald L. Wilson, Food and Drug Administration, Rockville, MD

Ronald H. Carlson, Health Resources and Services Administration, Rockville, MD

Craig Vanderwagen, Indian Health Service, Rockville, MD

John H. Ferguson, National Institutes of Health, Bethesda, MD

John T. Kalberer, Jr. (alternate), National Institutes of Health, Bethesda, MD

Edward Sondik, National Cancer Institute, National Institutes of Health, Bethesda, MD

Gregory J. Morosco, National Heart, Lung, and Blood Institute, National Institutes of Health, Bethesda, MD

Joan E. Blair, National Heart, Lung, and Blood Institute, National Institutes of Health, Bethesda, MD

Valerie Welsh, Office of Health Planning and Evaluation, Washington, DC

William A. Robinson, Office of Minority Health, Washington, DC

Robert A. Scholle, Office of Population Affairs, Washington, DC

Christine G. Spain, President's Council on Physical Fitness and Sports, Washington, DC

Other Members

Kathleen A. Loughrey, American Public Health Association, Washington, DC

Michael A. Stoto, Institute of Medicine, National Academy of Sciences, Washington, DC

Secretary's Council on Health Promotion and Disease Prevention

James O. Mason, *Chair*, Washington, DC

Edward N. Brandt, Jr., (Former Assistant Secretary for Health), Oklahoma City, OK

Stanley E. Broadnax, U.S. Conference of Local Health Officers, Cincinnati, OH

Theodore Cooper, (Former Assistant Secretary for Health), Kalamazoo, MI

Alan W. Cross, Association of Teachers of Preventive Medicine, Chapel Hill, NC

Gus T. Dalis, Association for the Advancement of Health Education, Downey, CA

Merlin K. Duval, (Former Assistant Secretary for Health), Phoenix, AZ

Charles C. Edwards, (Former Assistant Secretary for Health), LaJolla, CA

Roger O. Egeberg, (Former Assistant Secretary for Health), Rockville, MD

A. Garth Fisher, Provo, UT

Donald A. Henderson, Association of Schools of Public Health, Baltimore, MD

Joyce C. Lashof, Association of Schools of Public Health, Berkeley, CA

Philip R. Lee, (Former Assistant Secretary for Health), San Francisco, CA

Stephen H. Lipson, Indianapolis, IN

Joel L. Nitzkin, National Association of County Health Officials, New Orleans, LA

Kevin M. Patrick, Association of Teachers of Preventive Medicine, San Diego, CA

Thomas M. Vernon, Jr., Association of State and Territorial Health Officials, Denver, CO

Julius B. Richmond, (Former Assistant Secretary for Health), Boston, MA

Robert Rodale (deceased), Emmaus, PA

H. Denman Scott, Association of State and Territorial Health Officials, Providence, RI

F. Douglas Scutchfield, American College of Preventive Medicine, San Diego, CA

Bailus Walker, Jr., American Public Health Association, Oklahoma City, OK

Martin P. Wasserman, National Association of County Health Officials, Rockville, MD

Robert E. Windom, (Former Assistant Secretary for Health), Sarasota, FL

Committee on Health Objectives for the Year 2000, Institute of Medicine, National Academy of Sciences

Merlin K. Duval, *Chair*, Phoenix, AZ
Jack Elinson, Rutgers University, New Brunswick, NJ
Robert I. Levy, Sandoz Research Institute, East Hanover, NJ (until 5/88)
Anne Hubbard Mattson, Jefferson County Health Department, Birmingham, AL
Gilbert S. Omenn, University of Washington, Seattle, WA
Katharine Bauer Sommers, Institute of Medicine, Washington, DC

Institute of Medicine Staff

Samuel O. Thier, *President*
Michael A. Stoto, *Study Director*
Ruth Behrens
Enriqueta C. Bond
Marty Ellington
Gary B. Ellis
Kay C. Harris

Cynthia Howe
Roseanne Mctyre
Jane S. Durch
Connie Rosemont
Renie Schapiro
Donna D. Thompson

Coordinators of Priority Area Working Groups

Physical Activity and Fitness

Christine G. Spain, President's Council on Physical Fitness and Sports, Washington, DC

Nutrition

Darla E. Danford, National Institutes of Health (NIH), Bethesda, MD
Marilyn G. Stephenson, Center for Food Safety and Applied Nutrition, Food and Drug Administration (FDA), Washington, DC

Tobacco

Ronald M. Davis, Center for Chronic Disease Prevention and Health Promotion, Centers for Disease Control (CDC), Rockville, MD
John L. Bagrosky, Center for Chronic Disease Prevention, and Health Promotion (CDC), Rockville, MD

Alcohol and Other Drugs

Mary A. Jansen, Alcohol, Drug Abuse, and Mental Health Administration (ADAMHA), Rockville, MD

Family Planning

Robert A. Scholle, Office of Population Affairs, Washington, DC

Mental Health and Mental Disorders

Mary A. Jansen, Alcohol, Drug Abuse, and Mental Health Administration (ADAMHA), Rockville, MD

Violent and Abusive Behavior

James A. Mercy, Center for Environmental Health and Injury Control (CDC), Atlanta, GA
Mark L. Rosenberg, Center for Environmental Health and Injury Control (CDC), Atlanta, GA

Educational and Community-Based Programs

Dennis D. Tolsma, Centers for Disease Control, Atlanta, GA
Ronald H. Carlson, Health Resources and Services Administration (HRSA), Rockville, MD

Unintentional Injuries

J. Lee Annest, Center for Environmental Health and Injury Control (CDC), Atlanta, GA
Mark L. Rosenberg, Center for Environmental Health and Injury Control (CDC), Atlanta, GA

Occupational Safety and Health

Donald E. Ward, Jr., National Institute for Occupational Safety and Health (CDC), Atlanta, GA

129

Environmental Health

Daniel C. VanderMeer, National Institute of Environmental Health Sciences (NIH), Research Triangle Park, NC
Henry Falk, Center for Environmental Health and Injury Control (CDC), Atlanta, GA
Daniel A. Hoffman, Center for Environmental Health and Injury Control (CDC), Atlanta, GA

Food and Drug Safety

Ronald L. Wilson, Food and Drug Administration, Rockville, MD
I. David Wolfson, Food and Drug Administration, Rockville, MD

Oral Health

Helen C. Gift, National Institute of Dental Research (NIH), Bethesda, MD
Stephen B. Corbin, Center for Prevention Services (CDC), Bethesda, MD

Maternal and Infant Health

Ann M. Koontz, Maternal and Child Health Bureau (HRSA), Rockville, MD
Carol A. Delany, Maternal and Child Health Bureau (HRSA), Rockville, MD

Heart Disease and Stroke

Joan E. Blair, National Heart, Lung, and Blood Institute (NIH), Bethesda, MD

Cancer

Edward Sondik, National Cancer Institute (NIH), Bethesda, MD
Helen I. Meissner, National Cancer Institute (NIH), Bethesda, MD

Diabetes and Chronic Disabling Conditions

Benjamin T. Burton, National Institute of Diabetes and Digestive and Kidney Diseases (NIH), Bethesda, MD
James S. Marks, Center for Chronic Disease Prevention and Health Promotion (CDC), Atlanta, GA

HIV Infection

Jo Messore, National AIDS Program Office, Washington, DC

Sexually Transmitted Diseases

Willard Cates, Jr., Center for Prevention Services (CDC), Atlanta, GA
Stephen A. Morse, Center for Infectious Diseases (CDC), Atlanta, GA

Immunization and Infectious Diseases

Alan R. Hinman, Center for Prevention Services (CDC), Atlanta, GA
James M. Hughes, Center for Infectious Diseases (CDC), Atlanta, GA

Clinical Preventive Services

Ronald H. Carlson, Health Resources and Services Administration, Rockville, MD
Dennis D. Tolsma, Centers for Disease Control, Atlanta, GA

Surveillance and Data Systems

Ronald W. Wilson, National Center for Health Statistics (CDC), Hyattsville, MD
Patricia M. Golden, National Center for Health Statistics (CDC), Hyattsville, MD

Members of Priority Area Working Groups and Other Contributors

The following persons participated in development of the Healthy People 2000 objectives as members of working groups of professionals and in other significant roles. Many of them served on two or more working groups (as did a number of the priority area coordinators, who are not listed again).

Edgar Adams, National Institute on Drug Abuse (ADAMHA), Rockville, MD

Michael Adams, Center for Environmental Health and Injury Control (CDC), Atlanta, GA

David F. Adcock, University of South Carolina Medical School, Columbia, SC

Susan Addiss, Quinnipiack Valley Health District, Hamden, CT

J. Harrison Ager, National Institute of Diabetes and Digestive and Kidney Diseases (NIH), Bethesda, MD

E. Joseph Alderman, Georgia Department of Human Resources, Atlanta, GA

Caffilene Allen, Center for Infectious Diseases (CDC), Atlanta, GA

David Allen, Louisville and Jefferson County Health Department, Louisville, KY

Myron Allukian, Boston Department of Health and Hospitals, Boston, MA

Zili Amsel, National Institute on Drug Abuse (ADAMHA), Rockville, MD

Henry Anderson, Wisconsin Department of Health and Social Services, Madison, WI

Douglas L. Archer, Center for Food Safety and Applied Nutrition (FDA), Washington, DC

Katherine L. Armstrong, Western Consortium for Public Health, Berkeley, CA

Janet Arrowsmith, Food and Drug Administration, Rockville, MD

George Arsnow, Rehabilitation Services Administration, U.S. Department of Education, Washington, DC

Victor Avitto, Health Resources and Services Administration, Rockville, MD

Christine A. Bachrach, National Institute for Child Health and Human Development (NIH), Bethesda, MD

Shirley Bagley, National Institute on Aging (NIH), Bethesda, MD

Wendy Baldwin, National Institute for Child Health and Human Development (NIH), Bethesda, MD

Claudia Baquet, National Cancer Institute (NIH), Bethesda, MD

Robert Battjes, National Institute on Drug Abuse (ADAMHA), Rockville, MD

John A. Beare, Washington State Department of Social and Health Services, Olympia, WA

Robert W. Beck, Public Health Service, Rockville, MD

Christopher Benjamin, Office of Program Planning and Evaluation (CDC), Atlanta, GA

Heinz Berendes, National Institute of Child Health and Human Development (NIH), Bethesda, MD

Leonard Berg, Washington University School of Medicine, St. Louis, MO

Nancy Zinneman Berger, Association of State and Territorial Public Health Nutrition Program Directors, Hartford, CT

Lawrence Bergner, National Cancer Institute (NIH), Bethesda, MD

Betty Jo Berland, National Institute on Disability and Rehabilitation Research, U.S. Department of Education, Washington, DC

Darryl Bertolucci, National Institute on Alcohol Abuse and Alcoholism (ADAMHA), Rockville, MD

Richard M. Biery, Kansas City Health Department, Kansas City, MO

Rick Birkel, National Resource Center for Worksite Health Promotion, Washington, DC

Carl H. Blank, Training and Laboratory Program Office (CDC), Atlanta, GA

Joseph H. Blount, Center for Prevention Services (CDC), Atlanta, GA

John J. Boren, National Institute on Drug Abuse (ADAMHA), Rockville, MD

George Bouthilet, President's Committee on Mental Retardation, Washington, DC

Noble N. Bowie, National Highway Traffic Safety Administration, U.S. Department of Transportation (DOT), Washington, DC

Elizabeth Brannon, Health Resources and Services Adminisration, Rockville, MD

Albert Brasile, Center for Environmental Health and Injury Control (CDC), Atlanta, GA

George Brenneman, Indian Health Service, Rockville, MD

Ethel Briggs, National Council on the Handicapped, Washington, DC

Norma T. Brinkley-Staley, Health Resources and Services Administration, Rockville, MD

Martin Brown, National Cancer Institute (NIH), Bethesda, MD

Stuart T. Brown, DeKalb County Health Department, Decatur, GA

Georgia Buggs, Office of Minority Health, Washington, DC

William Bukoski, National Institute on Drug Abuse (ADAMHA), Rockville, MD

Thomas Burns, Indian Health Service, Rockville, MD

Richard Carnevale, Food Safety and Inspection Service, U.S. Department of Agriculture (USDA), Washington, DC

Judith L. Carpenter, Office of Intergovernmental Affairs, Washington, DC

Carl Caspersen, Center for Chronic Disease Prevention and Health Promotion (CDC), Atlanta, GA

Philip Chao, Food and Drug Administration, Rockville, MD

Bruce R. Chelikowsky, Indian Health Service, Rockville, MD

James Cleeman, National Heart, Lung, and Blood Institute (NIH), Bethesda, MD

Carolyn Clifford, National Cancer Institute (NIH), Bethesda, MD

Ronald F. Coene, National Center for Toxicological Research (FDA), Rockville, MD

Barbara Cohen, Office of Population Affairs, Washington, DC

Elaine Cohen, Health Resources and Services Administration, Rockville, MD

Mitchell L. Cohen, Center for Infectious Diseases (CDC), Atlanta, GA

J. Gary Collins, National Center for Health Statistics (CDC), Hyattsville, MD

Robert J. Collins, Indian Health Service, Rockville, MD

Eileen Connolly, Public Health Service—Region II, New York, NY

Gregory N. Connolly, Massachusetts Department of Public Health, Boston, MA

Frances Cotter, National Institute on Alcohol Abuse and Alcoholism (ADAMHA), Rockville, MD

Nancy F. Couey, Centers for Disease Control, Atlanta, GA

James F. Coyle, Federal Emergency Management Agency, Emmitsburg, MD

George Curlin, National Institute of Allergy and Infectious Diseases (NIH), Bethesda, MD

Dorynne Czechowicz, National Institute on Drug Abuse (ADAMHA), Rockville, MD

Anthony D'Angelo, Indian Health Service, Rockville, MD

Ada Davis, Bureau of Health Professions (HRSA), Rockville, MD

John Dement, National Institute of Environmental Health Sciences (NIH), Research Triangle Park, NC

Robert W. Denniston, Office for Substance Abuse Prevention (ADAMHA), Rockville, MD

Frank Destefano, Center for Chronic Disease Prevention and Health Promotion (CDC), Atlanta, GA

Terrence Donahue, Office of Justice Programs (DOT), Washington, DC

Denise Dougherty, Office of Technology Assessment, U.S. Congress, Washington, DC

Joseph S. Drage, National Institute of Neurological and Communicative Disorders and Stroke (NIH), Bethesda, MD

Frederick R. Drews, U.S. Army War College, Carlisle, PA

Peter Drotman, Center for Infectious Diseases (CDC), Atlanta, GA

Thomas F. Drury, National Institute of Dental Research (NIH), Bethesda, MD

Rosemary E. Duffy, U.S. Department of Veterans Affairs (VA), Washington, DC

Mary C. Dufour, National Institute on Alcohol Abuse and Alcoholism (ADAMHA), Rockville, MD

Allen B. Duncan, Food and Drug Administration, Rockville, MD

Thena M. Durham, Center for Prevention Services (CDC), Atlanta, GA

Spike Duzor, Health Care Financing Administration, Baltimore, MD

William W. Dyal, Public Health Program Practice Office (CDC), Atlanta, GA

Mark Eberhardt, National Center for Health Statistics (CDC), Hyattsville, MD

Brenda Edwards, National Cancer Institute (NIH), Bethesda, MD

Anita Eichler, National Institute of Mental Health (ADAMHA), Rockville, MD

Elaine Eklund, American Association of University Affiliated Programs for Persons with Developmental Disabilities, Silver Spring, MD

Pennifer Erickson, National Center for Health Statistics (CDC), Hyattsville, MD

Nancy D. Ernst, National Heart, Lung, and Blood Institute (NIH), Bethesda, MD

Joyce D. K. Essien, Public Health Program Practice Office (CDC), Atlanta, GA

David Evans, Agency for Toxic Substances and Disease Registry, Atlanta, GA

Vernard Evans, Administration on Developmental Disabilities, Office of Human Development Services (OHDS), Washington, DC

Ann Fainsinger, Alliance for Aging Research, Washington, DC

Mary E. Farmer, National Institute for Mental Health (ADAMHA), Rockville, MD

Marcia Fein, American Express, New York, NY

Michael C. Fiore, University of Wisconsin, Madison, WI

Michael Fishman, Maternal and Child Health Bureau (HRSA), Rockville, MD

Rebecca Fitch, Office of Special Education and Rehabilitation Services, U.S. Department of Education, Washington, DC

William FitzGerald, National Institute on Drug Abuse (ADAMHA), Rockville, MD

Allan L. Forbes, Rockville, MD

Willis R. Foster, National Institute of Diabetes and Digestive and Kidney Diseases (NIH), Bethesda, MD

Judith Fradkin, National Institute of Diabetes and Digestive and Kidney Diseases (NIH), Bethesda, MD

Dolores M. Franklin, Department of Human Services, Washington, DC

Paula Franklin, Office of Disability, Social Security Administration, Baltimore, MD

P. Jean Frazier, University of Minnesota, Minneapolis, MN

Frank J. Frodyma, Occupational Safety and Health Administration, U.S. Department of Labor (DOL), Washington, DC

Robinson Fulwood, National Heart, Lung, and Blood Institute (NIH), Bethesda, MD

Arthur S. Funke, Maternal and Child Health Bureau (HRSA), Rockville, MD

Lawrence J. Furman, Center for Prevention Services (CDC), Atlanta, GA

Judy Galloway, National Institute on Drug Abuse (ADAMHA), Rockville, MD

J. T. Garrett, Indian Health Service, Rockville, MD

Barbara Gerbert, University of California at San Francisco, San Francisco, CA

Martin Gerry, U.S. Department of Health and Human Services, Washington, DC

George M. Gillespie, Pan American Health Organization, Washington, DC

Evelyn Glass, Office of Population Affairs, Washington, DC

Tom Glynn, National Cancer Institute (NIH), Bethesda, MD

Dorothy Gohdes, Indian Health Service, Albuquerque, NM

Harold Goldsmith, National Institute of Mental Health (ADAMHA), Rockville, MD

Steve Gordon, National Institute of Arthritis and Musculoskeletal and Skin Diseases (NIH), Bethesda, MD

Peter Greenwald, National Cancer Institute (NIH), Bethesda, MD

Timothy W. Groza, National Institute for Occupational Safety and Health (CDC), Atlanta, GA

Antoinette Hagey, U.S. Department of Defense, Washington, DC

Carol Haines, National Heart, Lung, and Blood Institute (NIH), Bethesda, MD

Earl H. Handwerker, Center for Infectious Diseases (CDC), Atlanta, GA

Benjamin Hankey, National Cancer Institute (NIH), Bethesda, MD

Kevin S. Hardwick, Public Health Service, Rockville, MD

Thomas Harford, National Institute on Alcohol Abuse and Alcoholism (ADAMHA), Rockville, MD

William Harlan, National Heart, Lung, and Blood Institute (NIH), Bethesda, MD

Mary Harper, National Institute of Mental Health (ADAMHA), Rockville, MD

Peter Hartsock, National Institute on Drug Abuse (ADAMHA), Rockville, MD

Harry W. Haverkos, National Institute on Drug Abuse (ADAMHA), Rockville, MD

Barbara Hawkins, Indiana University, Bloomington, IN

Betty Hawks, Office of Minority Health, Washington, DC

Suzanne G. Haynes, National Cancer Institute (NIH), Bethesda, MD

Arlene P. Hegg, National Institute of Mental Health (ADAMHA), Rockville, MD

James T. Heimbach, Human Nutrition Information Service (USDA), Hyattsville, MD

Gerry Hendershot, National Center for Health Statistics (CDC), Hyattsville, MD

Kenneth L. Herrmann, Center for Infectious Diseases (CDC), Atlanta, GA

Stephen P. Heyse, National Institute of Arthritis and Musculoskeletal and Skin Diseases (NIH), Bethesda, MD

Penni St. Hilaire, Office of Intergovernmental Affairs, Rockville, MD

William Hiscock, Health Care Financing Administration, Baltimore, MD

Carol Hogue, Center for Chronic Disease Prevention and Health Promotion (CDC), Atlanta, GA

John Holland, National Defense University—Fort McNair, Washington, DC

John Holloszy, Washington University School of Medicine, St. Louis, MO

Janet Horan, Bureau of Health Professions (HRSA), Rockville, MD

Margorie C. Horn, National Center for Health Statistics (CDC), Hyattsville, MD

Philip R. Horne, Center for Prevention Services (CDC), Atlanta, GA

Constance Horner, U.S. Department of Health and Human Services, Washington, DC

Alice M. Horowitz, National Institute of Dental Research (NIH), Bethesda, MD

Vernon Houk, Center for Environmental Health and Injury Control (CDC), Atlanta, GA

Bettie Hudson, National Center for Health Statistics (CDC), Hyattsville, MD

Robert S. Hutchings, Center for Chronic Disease Prevention and Health Promotion (CDC), Rockville, MD
Karen Hymbaugh, Indian Health Service, Albuquerque, NM
George J. Jackson, Food and Drug Administration, Washington, DC
Jack Jackson, Center for Environmental Health and Injury Control (CDC), Atlanta, GA
Joyce Stokes Jackson, Health Care Financing Administration, Baltimore, MD
M. Yvonne Jackson, Indian Health Service, Rockville, MD
William R. Jarvis, Center for Infectious Diseases (CDC), Atlanta, GA
Patrick E. Johannes, Indian Health Service, Albuquerque, NM
Barry L. Johnson, Agency for Toxic Substances and Disease Registry, Atlanta, GA
Clifford Johnson, National Center for Health Statistics (CDC), Hyattsville, MD
Ernest W. Johnson, National Institute of Diabetes and Digestive and Kidney Diseases (NIH), Bethesda, MD
Sandie Johnson, Office for Substance Abuse Prevention (ADAMHA), Rockville, MD
Rhys Burton Jones, Wisconsin Division of Health, Madison, WI
James P. Kallenborn, Occupational Safety and Health Administration (DOL), Washington, DC
Glenn Kamber, Office for Treatment Improvement (ADAMHA), Rockville, MD
Robert Kane, University of Minnesota, Minneapolis, MN
George A. Kanuck, Office of Communication and Extramural Affairs (ADAMHA), Rockville, MD
Murray L. Katcher, Wisconsin Department of Health, Madison, WI
Wendy Kaye, Agency for Toxic Substances and Disease Registry (ATSDR), Atlanta, GA
Juliette S. Kendrick, Center for Chronic Disease Prevention and Health Promotion (CDC), Atlanta, GA
Miller H. Kerr, Centers for Disease Control, Atlanta, GA
Larry Kessler, National Cancer Institute (NIH), Bethesda, MD
Henry M. Kissman, National Library of Medicine, Bethesda, MD
Dushanka V. Kleinman, National Institute of Dental Research (NIH), Bethesda, MD
Joel Kleinman, National Center for Health Statistics (CDC), Hyattsville, MD
Robert N. Kohmescher, Center for Prevention Services (CDC), Atlanta, GA
Andrea Kopstein, National Institute on Drug Abuse (ADAMHA), Rockville, MD
John M. Korn, Jr., Center for Chronic Disease Prevention and Health Promotion (CDC), Atlanta, GA
Richard Kotomori, Indian Health Service, Rockville, MD
Nicholas Kozel, National Institute on Drug Abuse (ADAMHA), Rockville, MD
Marie Fanelli Kuczmarski, National Center for Health Statistics (CDC), Hyattsville, MD
George A. Kupfer, National Sanitation Foundation, Ann Arbor, MI
Thomas Lalley, National Institute of Mental Health (ADAMHA), Rockville, MD
Elizabeth Lambert, National Institute on Drug Abuse (ADAMHA), Rockville, MD
Garland Land, Missouri Department of Health, Jefferson City, MO
Elaine Lanza, National Cancer Institute (NIH), Bethesda, MD
Lynn A. Larsen, Center for Food Safety and Applied Nutrition (FDA), Washington, DC
Joyce Lazar, National Institute of Mental Health (ADAMHA), Rockville, MD
Bonnie Lee, Office of Health Affairs (FDA), Rockville, MD
Claude Lenfant, National Heart, Lung, and Blood Institute (NIH), Bethesda, MD
Bruce Leonard, Indian Health Service, Albuquerque, NM
Alan Leshner, National Institute on Mental Health (ADAMHA), Rockville, MD
Joel T. Levine, Health Resources and Services Administration, Rockville, MD
Luise Light, National Cancer Institute (NIH), Bethesda, MD
James A. Lipton, National Institute of Dental Research (NIH), Bethesda, MD
Barbara Lockhart, University of Iowa, Iowa City, IA
Beverly B. Long, National Prevention Coalition, Atlanta, GA
Gloriana M. Lopez, Bureau of Health Care Delivery and Assistance (HRSA), Rockville, MD
Max R. Lum, Office of External Affairs (ATSDR), Atlanta, GA
Geraldine Maccannon, Office of Minority Health, Washington, DC
Mark J. Magenheim, Sarasota County Public Health Unit, Sarasota, FL
Dolores M. Malvitz, Center for Prevention Services (CDC), Atlanta, GA
Ronald Manderscheid, National Institute of Mental Health (ADAMHA), Rockville, MD
Ann C. Maney, National Institute of Mental Health (ADAMHA), Rockville, MD
Michael Marge, National Commission on Disability, Syracuse University, Syracuse, NY
James Y. Marshall, American Dental Association, Chicago, IL

Carol A. Martin, Indian Health Service, Rockville, MD

Laura Y. Martin, Center for Environmental Health and Injury Control (CDC), Atlanta, GA

William J. Martone, Center for Infectious Diseases (CDC), Atlanta, GA

James Massey, National Center for Health Statistics (CDC), Hyattsville, MD

William J. Mayer, The Wyatt Company, Washington, DC

Robert McAlister, Association of State and Territorial Health Officials, McLean, VA

Sheila McCarthy, Maternal and Child Health Bureau (HRSA), Rockville, MD

Patrick McConnon, Center for Chronic Disease Prevention and Health Promotion (CDC), Atlanta, GA

George McCoy, Indian Health Service, City?

Sandra McElhaney, National Mental Health Association, Alexandria, VA

Steve Uranga McKane, Hartford Health Department, Hartford, CT

Jeffrey W. McKenna, National Cancer Institute (NIH), Bethesda, MD

John McKinlay, New England Research Institute, Watertown, MA

Mary McLean, Health Care Financing Administration, Washington, DC

Laura McNally, Health Resources and Financing Administration, Rockville, MD

Merle McPherson, Maternal and Child Health Bureau (HRSA), Rockville, MD

Robert E. Mecklenburg, Potomac, MD

Florence Meltzer, Office of Population Affairs, Washington, DC

Ronald B. Merrill, Health Resources and Services Administration, Rockville, MD

Walter Mertz, Human Nutrition Research Center (USDA), Beltsville, MD

Dorothy Meyer, Indian Health Service, Phoenix, AZ

C. Arden Miller, University of North Carolina at Chapel Hill, Chapel Hill, NC

William Modzeleski, U.S. Department of Education, Washington, DC

Judy Mohsberg, Office of Legislation and Policy (HCFA), Washington, DC

Mary Moien, National Center for Health Statistics (CDC), Hyattsville, MD

James M. Monroe, Center for Infectious Diseases (CDC), Atlanta, GA

Laura E. Montgomery, National Center for Health Statistics (CDC), Hyattsville, MD

John Moore, Center for Chronic Disease Prevention and Health Promotion (CDC), Atlanta, GA

Julian M. Morris, National Eye Institute (NIH), Bethesda, MD

James A. Mortimer, VA Medical Center, Minneapolis, MN

Eve K. Moscicki, National Institute of Mental Health (ADAMHA), Rockville, MD

Alanna Moshfegh, Human Nutrition Information Service (USDA), Hyattsville, MD

Doris Mosley, Health Resources and Services Administration, Rockville, MD

Barbara Nelson, National Institute for Occupational Safety and Health (CDC), Atlanta, GA

Gary Nelson, Centers for Disease Control, Atlanta, GA

Susan Newcomer, National Institute for Child Health and Human Development (NIH), Bethesda, MD

Linda C. Niessen, VA Medical Center, Perry Point, MD

Annette M. Nieves, Office of Minority Health, Washington, DC

Yuth Nimit, National Vaccine Program Office, Rockville, MD

Charles Q. North, Albuquerque Indian Hospital, Indian Health Service, Albuquerque, NM

Ruth Nowjack-Raymer, National Institute of Dental Research (NIH), Bethesda, MD

Godfrey P. Oakley, Jr., Center for Environmental Health and Injury Control (CDC), Atlanta, GA

Joanne Odenkirchen, National Cancer Institute (NIH), Bethesda, MD

Richard Olson, Indian Health Service, Rockville, MD

Walter A. Orenstein, Center for Prevention Services (CDC), Atlanta, GA

Marcia C. Ory, National Institute on Aging (NIH), Bethesda, MD

Donald C. Parks, Maternal and Child Health Bureau (HRSA), Rockville, MD

Sandra S. Parrino, National Commission on Disability, Briarcliff Manor, NY

Clifford H. Patrick, U.S. Department of Veteran Affairs, Durham, NC

Gregory Pawlson, George Washington University Medical Center, Washington, DC

Terry F. Pechacek, National Cancer Institute (NIH), Bethesda, MD

Marian Perlmutter, University of Michigan, Ann Arbor, MI

John P. Pierce, University of California, San Diego, La Jolla, CA

Anita Pikus, National Institute of Deafness and Other Communication Disorders (NIH), Bethesda, MD

Margaret Porter, Office of the Assistant Secretary for Planning and Evaluation, Washington, DC

Barry Portnoy, National Cancer Institute (NIH), Bethesda, MD

Curtis Posphisil, National Institute of Environmental Health Sciences (NIH), Research Triangle Park, NC
Arnold Potosky, National Cancer Institute (NIH), Bethesda, MD
Morris Potter, Center for Infectious Diseases (CDC), Atlanta, GA
Kenneth Powell, Center for Chronic Disease Prevention and Health Promotion (CDC), Atlanta, GA
William Pratt, National Center for Health Statistics (CDC), Hyattsville, MD
Ann E. Prendergast, Maternal and Child Health Bureau (HRSA), Rockville, MD
Philip Prorok, National Cancer Institute (NIH), Bethesda, MD
Glenn Provost, Center for Environmental Health and Injury Control (CDC), Atlanta, GA
James F. Quilty, Ohio Department of Public Health, Columbus, OH
Joan White Quinlan, Office for Substance Abuse Prevention (ADAMHA), Rockville, MD
Thomas C. Quinn, Johns Hopkins Hospital, Baltimore, MD
Amelie G. Ramirez, University of Texas Health Sciences Center at Houston, San Antonio, TX
Juan Ramos, National Institute of Mental Health (ADAMHA), Rockville, MD
David C. Ramsey, Center for Chronic Disease Prevention and Health Promotion (CDC), Atlanta, GA
Betty Reid, State Department of Education, Baltimore, MD
Nicholas P. Reuter, Food and Drug Administration, Rockville, MD
Peter H. Rheinstein, Center for Food Safety and Applied Nutrition (FDA), Rockville, MD
Carolyn Rimes, Office of the Actuary (HCFA), Baltimore, MD
Alice R. Ring, Centers for Disease Control, Atlanta, GA
Laverdia Roach, President's Committee on Mental Retardation, Washington, DC
David A. Robinson, National Heart, Lung, and Blood Institute (NIH), Bethesda, MD
Edward Roccella, National Heart, Lung, and Blood Institute (NIH), Bethesda, MD
Rose Mary Romano, Center for Chronic Disease Prevention and Health Promotion (CDC), Atlanta, GA
Joan Rosenbach, Health Resources and Services Administration, Rockville, MD
Harry Rosenberg, National Center for Health Statistics (CDC), Hyattsville, MD
Zeda Rosenberg, National Institute of Allergy and Infectious Diseases (NIH), Bethesda, MD
Louis Rossiter, Health Care Financing Administration, Washington, DC
Richard Rothenberg, Center for Chronic Disease Prevention and Health Promotion (CDC), Atlanta, GA
Charles Rothwell, National Center for Health Statistics (CDC), Hyattsville, MD
Kathy Roy, National Council on the Handicapped, Washington, DC
George W. Rutherford, Jr., U.S. Consumer Product Safety Commission, Washington, DC
Ruth Sanchez-Way, Office of Population Affairs, Washington, DC
Richard Sattin, Centers for Disease Control, Atlanta, GA
Steven L. Sauter, National Institute for Occupational Safety and Health (CDC), Atlanta, GA
James Scanlon, Office of Health Planning and Evaluation, Washington, DC
Charles Schade, American Public Health Association, Washington, DC
Peter C. Scheidt, National Institute for Child Health and Human Development (NIH), Bethesda, MD
Susan Schober, National Institute on Drug Abuse (ADAMHA), Rockville, MD
Edyth Schoenrich, The Johns Hopkins University, Baltimore, MD
Bettina Scott, Office for Substance Abuse Prevention (ADAMHA), Rockville, MD
Melvin Segal, Office for Substance Abuse Prevention (ADAMHA), Rockville, MD
Raymond Seltser, Agency for Health Care Policy and Research, Rockville, MD
Fred R. Shank, Center for Food Safety and Applied Nutrition (FDA), Washington, DC
Moira Shannon, National Center for Nursing Research (NIH), Bethesda, MD
Donald Shopland, National Cancer Institute (NIH), Bethesda, MD
Carl Shy, University of North Carolina at Chapel Hill, Chapel Hill, NC
Mervyn Silverman, American Foundation for AIDS Research, San Francisco, CA
Robert Silverman, National Institute of Diabetes and Digestive and Kidney Diseases (NIH), Bethesda, MD
John S. Small, National Institute of Dental Research (NIH), Bethesda, MD
Charles Smart, National Cancer Institute (NIH), Bethesda, MD
Richard J. Smith, Indian Health Service, Rockville, MD
Dixie E. Snider, Center for Prevention Services (CDC), Atlanta, GA
Harrison C. Spencer, Center for Infectious Diseases (CDC), Atlanta, GA
Jack N. Spencer, Center for Prevention Services (CDC), Atlanta, GA
Barry S. Stern, Bureau of Health Professions (HRSA), Rockville, MD
David Stevens, Bureau of Health Care Delivery and Assistance (HRSA), Rockville, MD

Dorothy Stephens, Health Resources and Services Administration, Rockville, MD

John A. Steward, Center for Environmental Health and Injury Control (CDC), Atlanta, GA

Deborah Jane Stokes, Association of Maternal and Child Health Programs, Gahanna, OH

Bob Stovenour, Administration on Developmental Disabilities (OHDS), Washington, DC

Nancy Stroup, Center for Environmental Health and Injury Control (CDC), Atlanta, GA

Linda A. Suydam, Center for Devices and Radiological Health (FDA), Rockville, MD

Elsie Taylor, National Institute on Alcohol Abuse and Alcoholism (ADAMHA), Rockville, MD

Glenn Taylor, Health Resources and Services Administration, Rockville, MD

William Taylor, Center for Environmental Health and Injury Control (CDC), Atlanta, GA

Steven Teutsch, Epidemiology Program Office (CDC), Atlanta, GA

J. Paul Thomas, National Institute on Disability and Rehabilitation Research, U.S. Department of Education, Washington, DC

Susan B. Toal, Centers for Disease Control, Atlanta, GA

Jerome Tobis, University of California Medical Center, Irvine, Orange, CA

Frederick T. Trowbridge, Center for Chronic Disease Prevention and Health Promotion (CDC), Atlanta, GA

Jeanne Trumble, Alcohol, Drug Abuse, and Mental Health Administration, Rockville, MD

Joan Van Nostrand, National Center for Health Statistics (CDC), Hyattsville, MD

Lyman Van Nostrand, Health Resources and Services Administration, Rockville, MD

Tina Vanderveen, National Institute on Drug Abuse (ADAMHA), Rockville, MD

Ecford Voit, National Institute of Mental Health (ADAMHA), Rockville, MD

Diane Wagener, National Center for Health Statistics (CDC), Hyattsville, MD

John B. Waller, Wayne State University, Detroit, MI

Larry Wannemacher, Health Resources and Services Administration, Rockville, MD

Nancy Wartow, Administration on Aging, (OHDS), Washington, DC

Judith N. Wasserheit, National Institute of Allergy and Infectious Diseases (NIH), Bethesda, MD

Nancy Watkins, Office of Program Planning and Evaluation (CDC), Atlanta, GA

Bill Weber, Bureau of Labor Statistics (DOL), Washington, DC

Linda Webster, Information Resource Management Office (CDC), Atlanta, GA

Jane A. Weintraub, University of North Carolina, Chapel Hill, NC

James A. Weixel, Food and Drug Administration, Rockville, MD

Thomas Wells, Utah Department of Health, Salt Lake City, UT

Janet Wetmore, National Institutes of Health, Bethesda, MD

Daniel F. Whiteside, Bureau of Resources Development (HRSA), Rockville, MD

Judith P. Wilkenfeld, Division of Advertising Practices, Federal Trade Commission, Washington, DC

James Willet, George Mason University, Fairfax, VA

T. Franklin Williams, National Institute on Aging (NIH), Bethesda, MD

Donna Wilson, National Institute for Occupational Safety and Health (CDC), Atlanta, GA

Deborah M. Winn, National Center for Health Statistics (CDC), Hyattsville, MD

Steven H. Woolf, Office of Disease Prevention and Health Promotion, Washington, DC

Marilyn Woolfolk, University of Michigan, Ann Arbor, MI

Catherine E. Woteki, Institute of Medicine, National Academy of Sciences, Washington, DC

James Young, President's Committee on Mental Retardation, Washington, DC

Jim F. Young, Administration on Children, Youth, and Families (OHDS), Washington, DC

K. Lum Young, Nebraska Department of Health, Lincoln, NE

Phyllis Zucker, Office of the Assistant Secretary for Planning and Evaluation, Washington, DC

Healthy People 2000 Consortium

National Organizations

Academy of General Dentistry

Aerobics and Fitness Association of America

Alcohol and Drug Problems Association of North America

Alliance for Aging Research

Alliance for Health

Amateur Athletic Union of the United States

American Academy of Child and Adolescent Psychiatry

American Academy of Family Physicians

American Academy of Ophthalmology

American Academy of Orthopaedic Surgeons

American Academy of Pediatric Dentistry

American Academy of Pediatrics

American Alliance for Health, Physical Education, Recreation, and Dance

American Art Therapy Association

American Association for Clinical Chemistry

American Association for Dental Research

American Association for Marriage and Family Therapy

American Association for Respiratory Care

American Association for the Advancement of Science

American Association of Certified Orthoptists

American Association of Colleges of Osteopathic Medicine

American Association of Colleges of Pharmacy

American Association of Dental Schools

American Association of Homes for the Aging

American Association of Occupational Health Nurses

American Association of Pathologists' Assistants

American Association of Public Health Dentistry

American Association of Public Health Physicians

American Association of Retired Persons

American Association of School Administrators

American Association of Suicidology

American Association of University Affiliated Programs for Persons with Developmental Disabilities

American Association on Mental Retardation

American Cancer Society

American College Health Association

American College of Cardiology

American College of Clinical Pharmacy

American College of Health Care Administrators

American College of Healthcare Executives

American College of Nurse-Midwives

American College of Nutrition

American College of Obstetricians and Gynecologists

American College of Occupational Medicine

American College of Physicians

American College of Preventive Medicine

American College of Radiology

American College of Sports Medicine

American Council on Alcoholism

American Dental Association

American Dental Hygienists' Association

American Diabetes Association

American Dietetic Association

American Federation of Teachers

American Geriatrics Society

American Heart Association

American Home Economics Association

American Hospital Association

American Indian Health Care Association

American Institute for Preventive Medicine

American Institute of Nutrition

American Kinesiotherapy Association

American Lung Association

American Meat Institute

American Medical Association

American Medical Student Association

American Nurses' Association

American Nutritionists Association

American Occupational Therapy Association

American Optometric Association

American Orthopaedic Society for Sports Medicine

American Osteopathic Academy of Sports Medicine

American Osteopathic Association

American Osteopathic Hospital Association

American Pharmaceutical Association

American Physical Therapy Association

American Physiological Society

American Podiatric Medical Association

American Psychiatric Association

American Psychiatric Nurses Association

American Psychological Association

American Public Health Association

American Red Cross

American Rehabilitation Counseling Association

American School Food Service Association

American School Health Association

American Social Health Association

American Society for Clinical Nutrition

American Society for Microbiology

American Society for Parenteral and Enteral Nutrition

American Society for Psycoprophylaxis in Obstetrics

American Society of Acupuncture

American Society of Addiction Medicine

American Society of Allied Health Professions

American Society of Hospitai Pharmacists

American Society of Human Genetics

American Society of Ocularists

American Speech-Language-Hearing Association

American Spinal Injury Association

American Statistical Association

American Thoracic Society

Arthritis Foundation

Asian American Health Forum

Association for Applied Psychophysiology and Biofeedback

Association for Fitness in Business

Association for Hospital Medical Education

Association for Practitioners in Infection Control

Association for Retarded Citizens of the United States

Association for the Advancement of Automotive Medicine

Association for the Advancement of Health Education

Association for Vital Records and Health Statistics

Association of Academic Health Centers

Association of American Indian Physicians

Association of American Medical Colleges

Association of Clinical Scientists

Association of Community Health Nursing Educators

Association of Food and Drug Officials

Association of Maternal and Child Health Programs

Association of Pediatric Oncology Nurses

Association of Rehabilitation Nurses

Association of Schools of Public Health

Association of State and Territorial Dental Directors

Association of State and Territorial Directors of Nursing

Association of State and Territorial Directors of Public Health Education

Association of State and Territorial Health Officials

Association of State and Territorial Public Health Laboratory Directors

Association of State and Territorial Public Health Nutrition Directors

Association of State and Territorial Public Health Social Work

Association of Teachers of Preventive Medicine

Association of Technical Personnel in Ophthalmology

Black Congress on Health, Law, and Economics

Blue Cross and Blue Shield Association

Boys Scouts of America

Business Roundtable

Camp Fire

Cardiovascular Credentialing International/National Board of Cardiovascular Technology

Catholic Health Association of the United States

Children's Hospital National Medical Center

College of American Pathologists

Council for Responsible Nutrition

Council of Medical Specialty Societies

Dairy and Food Nutrition Council of the Southeast

Emergency Nurses Association

Eye Bank Association of America

Federation of American Societies for Experimental Biology

Federation of Nurses and Health Professionals

Food Marketing Institute

Future Homemakers of America

Gerontological Society of America

Girl Scouts of the United States of America

Great Lakes Association of Clinical Medicine

Grocery Manufacturers of America

Group Health Association of America

Health Industry Manufacturers Association

Health Insurance Association of America

Highway Users Federation for Safety and Mobility

Institute of Food Technologists

International Association for Enterostomal Therapy

International Lactation Consultant Association

International Life Sciences Institute

International Patient Education Council

La Leche League International

Learning Disabilities Association of America

March of Dimes Birth Defects Foundation

Maternal and Child Health Network

Maternity Center Association

Midwives' Alliance of North America

Migrant Clinicians Network

Mothers Against Drunk Driving

NAACOG—The Organization of Obstetric, Gynecologic, and Neonatal Nurses

NARD—formerly National Association of Retail Druggists

National AIDS Network

National Alliance for the Mentally Ill

National Alliance of Black School Educators

National Alliance of Nurse Practitioners

National Association for Hispanic Elderly

National Association for Home Care

National Association for Human Development

National Association for Music Therapy

National Association for Sport and Physical Education

National Association of Biology Teachers

National Association of Childbearing Centers

National Association of Community Health Centers

National Association of Counties

National Association of County Health Officials

National Association of Elementary School Principals

National Association of Governors Councils on Physical Fitness and Sports

National Association of Neonatal Nurses

National Association of Optometrists and Opticians

National Association of Pediatric Nurse Associates and Practitioners

National Association of RSVP Directors

National Association of School Nurses

National Association of Secondary School Principals

National Association of Social Workers

National Association of State Alcohol and Drug Abuse Directors

National Association of State Boards of Education

National Association of State NET Program Coordinators

National Association of State School Nursing Consultants

National Black Nurses Association

National Board of Medical Examiners

National Center for Health Education

National Coalition of Hispanic Health and Human Services Organization

National Commission Against Drunk Driving

National Committee for Adoption

National Committee for Prevention of Child Abuse

National Conference of State Legislatures

National Consumers League

National Council for International Health

National Council for the Education of Health Professionals in Health Promotion

National Council on Alcoholism and Drug Dependence

National Council on Disability
National Council on Health Laboratory Services
National Council on Patient Information and
    Education
National Council on Self-Help and Public Health
National Council on the Aging
National Dairy Council
National Environmental Health Association
National Extension Homemakers Council
National Family Planning and Reproductive Health
    Association
National Federation of State High School
    Associations
National Food Processors Association
National Head Injury Foundation
National Health Council
National Health Lawyers Association
National Hearing Aid Society
National Institute for Fitness and Sport
National Kidney Foundation
National League for Nursing
National Lesbian and Gay Health Foundation
National Medical Association
National Mental Health Association
National Museum of Health and Medicine
National Nurses Society on Addictions
National Organization for Women
National Organization on Adolescent Pregnancy and
    Parenting
National Osteoporosis Foundation
National Pest Control Association
National Pressure Ulcer Advisory Panel
National PTA
National Recreation and Park Association
National Safety Council
National School Boards Association

National Society of Allied Health
National Society to Prevent Blindness
National Strength and Conditioning Association
National Stroke Association
National Wellness Institute
National Women's Health Network
NEA Health Information Network
Nursing Network on Violence Against Women
Oncology Nursing Society
Paralyzed Veterans of America
People's Medical Society
Pharmaceutical Manufacturers Association
Planned Parenthood Federation of America
Population Association of America
Produce Marketing Association
Salt Institute
Salvation Army
Society for Nutrition Education
Society for Public Health Education
Society of Behavioral Medicine
Society of Hospital Epidemiologists of America
Society of Prospective Medicine
Society of State Directors of Health, Physical
    Education, and Recreation
South Cove Community Health Center
State Family Planning Administrators
United States Chamber of Commerce
United States Conference of Mayors
United Way of America
Visiting Nurse Associations of America
Voluntary Hospitals of America
Washington Business Group on Health
Wellness Councils of America—WELCOA
Western Consortium for Public Health
Women's Sports Foundation

State and Territorial Health Departments

Alabama	Kansas	North Dakota
Alaska	Kentucky	Ohio
American Samoa	Louisiana	Oklahoma
Arizona	Maine	Oregon
Arkansas	Maryland	Pennsylvania
California	Massachusetts	Puerto Rico
Colorado	Michigan	Rhode Island
Connecticut	Minnesota	South Carolina
Delaware	Mississippi	South Dakota
District of Columbia	Missouri	Tennessee
Florida	Montana	Texas
Georgia	Nebraska	Utah
Guam	Nevada	Vermont
Hawaii	New Hampshire	Virginia
Idaho	New Jersey	Washington
Illinois	New Mexico	West Virginia
Indiana	New York	Wisconsin
Iowa	North Carolina	Wyoming

C. Priority Area Lead Agencies

1.	Physical Activity and Fitness	President's Council on Physical Fitness and Sports
2.	Nutrition	National Institutes of Health Food and Drug Administration
3.	Tobacco	Centers for Disease Control
4.	Alcohol and Other Drugs	Alcohol, Drug Abuse, and Mental Health Administration
5.	Family Planning	Office of Population Affairs
6.	Mental Health and Mental Disorders	Alcohol, Drug Abuse, and Mental Health Administration
7.	Violent and Abusive Behavior	Centers for Disease Control
8.	Educational and Community-Based Programs	Centers for Disease Control Health Resources and Services Administration
9.	Unintentional Injuries	Centers for Disease Control
10.	Occupational Safety and Health	Centers for Disease Control
11.	Environmental Health	National Institutes of Health Centers for Disease Control
12.	Food and Drug Safety	Food and Drug Administration
13.	Oral Health	National Institutes of Health Centers for Disease Control
14.	Maternal and Infant Health	Health Resources and Services Administration
15.	Heart Disease and Stroke	National Institutes of Health
16.	Cancer	National Institutes of Health
17.	Diabetes and Chronic Disabling Conditions	National Institutes of Health Centers for Disease Control
18.	HIV Infection	National AIDS Program Office
19.	Sexually Transmitted Diseases	Centers for Disease Control
20.	Immunization and Infectious Diseases	Centers for Disease Control
21.	Clinical Preventive Services	Health Resources and Services Administration Centers for Disease Control
22.	Surveillance and Data Systems	Centers for Disease Control

Index to Summary List of Objectives

The Jones and Bartlett Series in Health Sciences